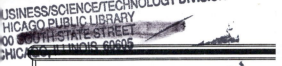

Lillian R. Brazin, MS, AHIP

The Guide to Complementary and Alternative Medicine on the Internet

Pre-publication
REVIEWS,
COMMENTARIES,
EVALUATIONS . . .

"As a physician trained in alleopathic medicine with more than a passing interest in complementary therapies, I welcome this book. The Internet has made available all sorts of information to the public at large—much of it good, and unfortunately, much of it ill-informed and potentially dangerous. This book identifies Web sites with known track records, provides a basic primer in searching the Internet, and offers helpful guidance in filtering and evaluating the quality of the information provided.

I believe that knowledge is powerful, and that well-informed consumers will continue to drive improvements in the quality of the health care they receive. This book provides the general public with some of the tools they will need to avoid unproven therapies and improve their lives.

I found *The Guide to Complementary and Alternative Medicine on the Internet* well organized, easy to read, and full of useful tips for Web browsers on subjects within and outside the realm of complementary therapies."

Kenneth Mikio Ogawa, DMD, MD
Board Certified, American Academy of Family Practice; Member, American Academy of Medical Acupuncture

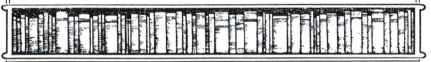

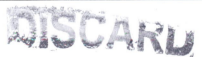

"Finally, a reputable guide to the often confusing maze of complementary and alternative medicine information available on the Internet! A well-written, easy to follow style that will guide even the most inexperienced Web users to the information they are seeking and encourage them to ask questions before making vital decisions affecting their well-being. In our current health care environment it is important that patients seek information on their own and feel in control. I feel very comfortable recommending this book to patients for aid in their quest for knowledge. Readers will appreciate the book's open yet cautionary approach toward sites that not only provide information but sell products as well.

I particularly enjoyed the sections on nutrition, diabetes, herbal medicine, and GI disorders as these are topics I get asked about most frequently in my profession. Many of the recommended sites are now in my favorite places folder on my computer!"

Beth E. Schwartzman, RD, LDN, CDE
Registered Dietician,
Certified Diabetes Educator
at Albert Einstein Medical Center

"This is a great and timely reference for 'real people' interested in finding out more about complementary and alternative medicine. It is clear, practical, well organized, and easy to read. The glossary of terms is especially useful for the newcomer to this field. Brazin stresses the importance of checking with a physician, and knowing and researching, as she has done, your Internet sites. Her insights and comments make this book interesting as she takes you from herbal cancer treatments to pet therapies. Brushing a pet may be one of the best complementary medicines around! As a small animal veterinarian for thirteen years, I add many nutritional and physical therapies to my standard protocols. Clients are asking more and more for something else to do, both for themselves and their pets. This book would be a useful addition to any library."

Jacqueline H. Menninger, VMD
Owner, The Family Pet Clinic PC,
Southampton, PA

More pre-publication
REVIEWS, COMMENTARIES, EVALUATIONS . . .

The Haworth Information Press®
An Imprint of The Haworth Press
New York • London • Oxford

The Guide
to Complementary
and Alternative Medicine
on the Internet

THE HAWORTH INFORMATION PRESS
Internet Guides to Consumer Health Care
M. Sandra Wood, MLS
Editor

The Guide to Complementary and Alternative Medicine on the Internet by Lillian R. Brazin

Internet Guide to Travel Health by Elizabeth Conner

The Guide
to Complementary
and Alternative Medicine
on the Internet

Lillian R. Brazin, MS, AHIP

The Haworth Information Press®
An Imprint of The Haworth Press
New York • London • Oxford

Published by

The Haworth Information Press®, an imprint of The Haworth Press, Inc., 10 Alice Street, Binghamton, NY 13904-1580.

TR: 3.15.04

PUBLISHER'S NOTE
Due to the ever-changing nature of the Internet, Web site names and addresses, though verified to the best of the publisher's ability, should not be accepted as accurate without independent verification.

Cover design by Marylouise E. Doyle.

Library of Congress Cataloging-in-Publication Data

Brazin, Lillian R.
    The guide to complementary and alternative medicine on the Internet / Lillian R. Brazin.
      p. cm.
    Includes bibliographical references and index.
    ISBN 0-7890-1570-6 (hardcover : alk. paper)—ISBN 0-7890-1571-4 (softcover : alk. paper)
    1. Alternative medicine—Computer network resources—Directories. I. Title.
R733.B795 2003
025.06'6155—dc21
                                                     2003012258

To Fudge, Truffles, and Maxine
who provide pet therapy to their mistress

ABOUT THE AUTHOR

Lillian R. Brazin, MS, AHIP, is Director of Library Services at the Albert Einstein Healthcare Network in Philadelphia. She has over thirty years of experience as a medical reference librarian, working in the areas of online services, user instruction, and management of academic health sciences libraries. She has eight years of experience as an evening and weekend reference librarian for the Free Library of Philadelphia. Ms. Brazin has published numerous articles and developed and taught workshops on Internet resources. She is a member of the Academy of Health Information Professionals (Distinguished Level), American Library Association, Medical Library Association, and Special Libraries Association.

CONTENTS

Preface

My personal experiences with complementary and alternative medicine (CAM) began in graduate (library) school when I worked as an assistant at a psychiatric research laboratory. The medical school-affiliated laboratory conducted research on hypnosis and biofeedback (relaxation) training, among other subjects. These therapies were studied as aids to pain control.

My late husband was an old-time family doctor, an osteopathic general practitioner who "adjusted" my neck on our first date. He once tried a patient's ethnic family recipe for boiled gingerroot in an attempt to relieve my migraine headaches. Even now I gag at the taste of ginger!

Recently, I have used (with some success) supplements of riboflavin, choline, vitamin B_6, and vitamin E to lessen the frequency of migraine headaches. Friends use acupuncture, echinacea, soy milk, and evening primrose oil for a variety of ills.

As a librarian who has worked in U.S. hospitals, medical schools, and public libraries for over three decades, I have noticed a growing acceptance of and interest in the field of complementary and alternative medicine by both the general public and health professionals such as doctors and nurses. Sometimes called integrative medicine, CAM generally refers to philosophies of treating illnesses and approaches to the patient that are not commonly considered by Western (traditional or mainstream) medicine. Technically, complementary therapy differs from alternative medicine. The former refers to therapy used together with traditional (Western) medicine, while the latter term refers to therapy used in place of mainstream medicine. Integrative medicine/therapy has a meaning similar to complementary therapy in that it refers to treatments used in conjunction with

Western medicine, utilizing whatever methods are most effective without favoring one system over another (traditional or alternative).

Many books and Web sites about complementary and alternative medicine tout the field with an enthusiasm bordering on religious fervor. The most popular authors in the field all seem to be charismatic guru types with piercing eyes. I, however, have a conservative perspective on the subject. Neutrality and caution are my watchwords because I have seen so many health fads and beliefs change or fall out of favor over time. For nearly a decade I have also worked in public libraries and have had the opportunity to listen to the health concerns of people from many cultures. Depending on their age, ethnic background, health status, economic circumstances, profession, and sex, people have different attitudes toward their bodies and toward the medical establishment (doctors, nurses, medical insurers). Some individuals are comfortable using computers; some are not. Not everyone has a home computer. Some prefer to leave decisions concerning their health to health practitioners. Some may want to take charge of their own health treatment. People have different methods of seeking health information. Some people are shy about asking for help, while others are very assertive. This book is aimed primarily at those readers who have just begun to explore the Internet, who are shy about talking with friends, relatives, and doctors about medical issues. I hope you look at the Internet as a new world of adventure that you can travel to from the safety and anonymity of your home. Enjoy!

Acknowledgments

The many dedicated physicians, nurses, dietitians, and therapists at the Albert Einstein Healthcare Network are to be commended for embracing CAM practices for their patients and themselves. I especially wish to acknowledge my own primary physicians, Drs. B and Z, who are always open to new practices, both traditional and complementary. My veterinarian, Dr. M, is equally knowledgeable and eager to accept new theories and treatments. Last, I thank my editor, Sandy Wood, for her encouragement and patience.

Chapter 1

Words of Wisdom

INTRODUCTION

Have you noticed that many health insurers now routinely cover acupuncture, chiropractic manipulation, yoga, and massage? Most medical schools and hospitals are establishing centers for integrative medicine and adding CAM courses to the medical school curriculum. Hospitals offer massages, yoga, Feldenkrais, tai chi, and pain control instruction to employees, patients, and the general public. Americans have embraced CAM in growing numbers. In 1993 a report in the *New England Journal of Medicine*[1] revealed startling statistics: in the United States more visits were made to alternative medicine practitioners than to family doctors. Insurance paid for only one-fourth of these expenditures. A study published in *Journal of the American Medical Association (JAMA)* in 1998[2] showed that more than 42 percent of Americans who responded to a survey said they had used an alternative medical therapy. The therapies they used most often were herbal medicine, massage, megavitamins, self-help groups, folk remedies, energy healing, and homeopathy. They reported spending more than $27 billion in 1997, more than was spent out of pocket for hospitalizations in the United States.

Americans are using CAM treatments in various ways: as an alternative to conventional/traditional therapies or as additions to such treatments (complementary or integrative approaches).

What types of people use CAM? They tend to be well read, well educated, and suffering from chronic or terminal conditions. They embrace CAM not necessarily because they are dissatisfied with Western medicine or their health practitioners but because they view some CAM practices as reflecting their own beliefs toward health and their personal values and lifestyles. Widely publicized deaths and birth defects caused by prescription medications add to the popularity of "natural" remedies.

More than half of U.S. physicians reported using for themselves (or recommending for their patients) some CAM therapies.[3] Although these cited articles are several years old, from the proliferation of books, magazines, videos, Web sites, and general newspaper articles on CAM, we can be pretty sure that CAM has caught on with the average American in a big way. Within this trend, we should not forget the influence of personal computers (PCs). Consumers can research health topics without visiting the library. The Internet, which includes Web sites, online discussion groups, chat rooms, newsgroups, and more, allows people to present information to the world with an immediacy (and lack of censorship) not generally available with other forms of expression. This is a blessing and a problem; there is so much information and it is difficult to evaluate. This book will help you choose the best CAM sites for your needs.

HOW I SELECTED THESE WEB SITES

So many Web sites, so little time.

I made selections based on criteria many health and information experts have written about in newspaper and magazine articles: the author's or organization's expertise, ease of use, currency, lack of bias or commercialism, accuracy, and respect for privacy. For this book I limited listings to sites primarily from North America. My search strategies included keyword searches on several search engines, but I also explored the "preselected" Web sites in search engine directories and university library Web sites. Government Web sites were useful and often led me to additional resources. Recommendations in newspapers, both national and local, and popular magazines added to my selections. I spoke with medical librarian colleagues and recalled the sites that had been most helpful answering the questions of my library users. Finally, I referred to my own stash of favorite CAM resources on the Internet—the sites I have "bookmarked" on my computer at home. You can bookmark your own favorites, using these selections as a starting point.

WHY READ THIS BOOK?

> The beginning of health is to know the disease.
>
> Spanish proverb

I teach classes for women about finding and evaluating health information on the Internet. The Internet can be frightening and overwhelming because there is so much information to sift through, digest, and evaluate. The different chapters of this book will help you identify the Internet CAM resources you can trust. The book will clarify questions and controversial topics such as the following:

- How can you be certain that the information you find is correct?
- How do you locate a Web site that was recommended to you?
- How do you begin to research a particular health problem?
- What is the Pilates exercise method that Jacqueline Kennedy Onassis helped popularize in the 1960s? It is trendy again. There are Pilates studios in most major cities.

- Your supermarket sells St. John's wort, gingko biloba, and vitamins A through Z. Should you take soy supplements for hot flashes?
- What is the meaning of dot com, edu, gov, mailing lists, :), BTW, LOL, flames, Netiquette, etc.?

Warning: This book is not a substitute for advice and recommendations from your doctor or other health care provider. Always share your concerns, as well as any Internet or print health information, with your health care provider before you make any changes regarding treatment or lifestyle. Even seemingly harmless diet supplements, for example, can interact with prescribed medications and have dangerous results. Your physician needs to know your entire medication history (prescribed medications as well as over-the-counter potions) to treat you properly. In the long run, you will really achieve better results if you adopt a team approach with your doctor. A health practitioner should first evaluate all symptoms.

If you think your family doctor will laugh when you suggest CAM treatments, you might be surprised. The medical journals most commonly read by doctors *(JAMA, New England Journal of Medicine, The Lancet,* and *Canadian Medical Association Journal)* feature articles on CAM. The U.S. federal government takes it seriously enough to have established a dozen centers throughout the country to research evidence that CAM therapies are truly effective. Partner with your doctor. Show him or her the articles you read in *Time, Newsweek,* and *The New York Times.* Speak with your local public librarian. Most public libraries contain up-to-date books on health topics, including CAM, and librarians can show you how to research topics on the Internet and on electronic groupings of databases such as InfoTrac and OVID to which many public libraries subscribe.

Another warning: The Internet is dynamic—it changes constantly. Web sites are removed. Sites move to new "addresses" (http://www . . .) and do not always leave a forwarding address. A site may be abandoned, and its information may become outdated. Links within a Web site may go nowhere. Names of Internet resources may change or the authors may change. At the time this book was submitted for publication, all Web addresses and names of sites were correct.

LET THE SEARCHER BEWARE: THE GOOD, THE BAD, AND THE UGLY— EVALUATING CAM WEB SITES

A fool believes everything.

Traditional proverb

Would you take medical advice from a sixteen-year-old? A popular magazine posed this question to its readers. It may sound silly, but unless you keep some guidelines in mind when surfing the Net, you might find yourself looking at a colorful Web site that is full of incorrect, biased, or even dangerous information. Anyone can create an attractive Web site that appears to be authoritative—even your teenaged neighbor. The following should be evident on good sites:

- *The identity of the creator:* Is the person or group responsible for the content readily identified? Can you contact them (e-mail, telephone, fax, or mail)? What are the credentials of the creator (education, experience, affiliation, and publications)?
- *Currency:* When was the site last updated? Are all the links to other Web sites still "live" (working)? Is the site frequently "down" for maintenance?
- *Seal of approval:* Has a national health organization or the federal government recommended the site? Does it bear the "HONCode" logo? (This code is awarded to sites that meet the HONCode of Conduct). See **Health on the Net**

Foundation (HON) (http://www.hon.ch/). This group was created in 1995 and is an international Swiss organization. Its mission is to guide Internet searchers to reliable and useful online medical and health information. It sets ethical standards for those who develop health and medical Web sites. The HON site can also be searched by keyword to locate approved sites that have been categorized as educational, commercial, or individual.

Another health Web site accrediting organization is **URAC** (http://websiteaccreditation.urac.org/). URAC's motto is "Quality health Web sites you can trust." URAC, also known as the American Accreditation Healthcare Commission, is a nonprofit charitable organization founded in 1990 with the goal to establish standards for the health care industry. According to their Web site, URAC's mission is "to promote continuous improvement in the quality and efficiency of healthcare delivery by achieving a common understanding of excellence . . . through the establishment of standards . . . and a process of accreditation." As of May 2003, forty-three sites have URAC accreditation, including **MEDLINEplus** (http://www.medlineplus.gov). URAC aims to help consumers identify sites that meet high accountability and quality standards. URAC lists the accredited Web sites with the name of the company that produces the site. The sites are reviewed annually, and the date the accreditation expires is listed. Under URAC's "Health Web Site Accreditation Program," sites are evaluated for disclosure of financial backing and sponsorship, privacy and security, and quality and oversight standards.

For a good guide to determining a CAM (or other health) site's credibility or the validity of its claims, check out **Quackwatch** (http://www.quackwatch.com). This site, however, sometimes takes a negative view toward CAM therapies. Quackwatch is excellent for exposing fraudulent therapies and devices. Another site to visit for information on medical fraud is the **National Council Against Health Fraud** (http://www.ncahf.org). It is a good source for breaking news items. Health professionals write the articles.

- *Bias:* Is the site selling products such as vitamins, books, and equipment? Is the site produced or sponsored by a drug company? Does the site advertise a practitioner's clinic?
- *Purpose:* Is the purpose of the Web site clearly indicated? Is it meant to educate, inform, support, sell something, or attract customers or patients?
- *Audience:* Who is the intended audience: CAM professionals (therapists, physicians, instructors), medical professionals, or consumers?
- *Attractiveness of the site:* Is it easy to use and pleasing to the eye?
- *Origin:* Are you the master of your *domain*? The two- or three-letter tag at the end of a Web site address (gov, edu, com, org) indicates the origin of the site. The "gov" domain means you have found a government Web site, "edu" is an educational institution such as a school or hospital, "com" is a business, and "org" is an organization. More domains are under consideration. Sometimes an abbreviation follows the domain to indicate a foreign language or country ("uk" is the United Kingdom, "fr" is France, "esp" is Spain or Spanish language). Web sites in the "gov" or "edu" domains have the most credibility. When in doubt, choose one of these sites.

Finally, try to familiarize yourself with several general CAM Web sites, in case your favorite site disappears. Most of the government and academic sites are kept up to date. Keep your eyes open when reading the newspaper or your favorite general news magazine – all are great sources for learning about new medical and CAM Web sites.

GETTING STARTED

No one is without knowledge except he who asks no questions.

African proverb

Before you begin to research complementary and alternative treatments, you should be certain you are knowledgeable about traditional therapies and the causes, course, and prognosis (future outcome) of your illness or symptoms. Are you aware of new drugs, procedures, and basic medical knowledge concerning your condition? Do you know what is in the research "pipeline"? Are there "centers of excellence" for treating your condition in your community? Have you had a heart-to-heart chat with your health care providers about your condition and the progress you are making in dealing with it? Have you told your health care providers that you are ready to explore CAM? If you have done all of these things, you are ready to begin to explore CAM Internet resources.

First look at government resources, starting with **MED-LINEplus** (Medlineplus.gov). You will find dozens of diseases at this site, along with a medical dictionary, directories, diagrams, and links to government agencies and national health organizations. Some of these traditional medical sites include information about approved and nonapproved CAM therapies and have their own online discussion/support groups.

The next step is to visit Internet sites for national disease societies and organizations. Some, such as the **National Osteoporosis Foundation** (http://www.nof.org) and the **Leukemia and Lymphoma Society** (http://www.leukemia.org), include the text of pamphlets or information about research currently being conducted.

Now check out the sites developed by universities (usually libraries) and public library groups. These sites generally include only those Web resources that meet criteria for currency, accuracy, etc. Move on to Internet sites dealing with specific thera-pies, such as herbal medicine, hypnosis, Rolfing, massage, and acupuncture.

Last, try search engines to locate other sites. Search by key-word, phrase, name of practitioner, symptom, and disease. Use the quality criteria discussed previously. Show the Web sites to your health practitioner. Never put anything into or on your body (pills, liquids, oils, ointments, inhalants) without telling your health practitioner what you plan to do. Do not begin exer-cise regimens before having a medical checkup. *Do not stop* your traditional therapy without discussing this with your health practitioner.

After beginning any CAM treatment, stop immediately and call your health practitioner if any new pain or other symptoms develop. Natural ingredients are not necessarily nonallergenic or benign (harmless).

Use common sense: if coffee enemas seem bizarre to you, do not let yourself be persuaded otherwise! Do you really believe that the color of your eyes affects your health? Does a diet of one food or only liquids sound healthy to you? Be smart about this—it is your health and your life we are talking about. Now, let's begin!

NETIQUETTE

Because it is so easy to dash off a message over the Internet, some of us forget basic rules of etiquette, grammar, and spell-ing. Also, some features are unique to the Internet. Here are some words of advice:

- Do not divulge personal information when posting to a group (whether a mailing list, bulletin board, chat room, or online support group). Messages may be stored (archived) or made available to the public.

- Do not forward messages from other people without first obtaining their permission.
- Do not type in all capital letters. This is annoying and is known as "shouting."
- Do not send replies in a fit of anger.
- Do not insult ("flame") someone over the Internet.
- Do not stalk or harass others in cyberspace. Carefully consider the impression your message leaves. (Could your words be misunderstood as insulting or insensitive?)
- Do not clog up mailboxes by posting "me too" messages. As a rule, do not reply or post a message unless you have a new or unique opinion to add.
- Reply to individuals, rather than to the entire group, when appropriate.
- Do not be embarrassed to state that you are a "newbie" (newcomer) to discussion lists.
- Do not be afraid to "lurk" for a while (read but not post messages) when you first join a discussion group. It takes a while to get a feel for the "culture" of the group.
- Do not overdo emoticons (the punctuation marks people use to express emotion in e-mail) or acronyms (abbreviations in which each letter stands for initials of each word). Examples of emoticons and acronyms follow:

  :(sad
  :) happy
  lol laughing out loud
  rotfl rolling on the floor laughing
  btw by the way
  THX thanks
  %-) confused
  FAQ frequently asked questions

  For more emoticons and abbreviations, see **Acronyms, Emoticons and Smilies Page** (http://www.Muller-Godschalk. com/emoticon.html).

- Follow the rules at work. Some companies have very strict rules about appropriate use of the Internet and e-mail. Many companies monitor employees' messages and Internet surfing. When in doubt, use a home computer. It is not worth losing your job over this!

NOTES

1. Eisenberg, D.M., Kessler, R.C., Foster, C., Norlock, F.E., Calkins, D.R., and Delbanco, T.L. (1993). Unconventional Medicine in the United States: Prevalence, Costs, and Patterns of Use. *New England Journal of Medicine* 328: 246-252.

2. Eisenberg, D.M., Davis, R.B., Ettner, S.L., Appel, S., Wilkey, S., Van Rompay, M., and Kessler, R.C. (1998). Trends in Alternative Medicine Use in the United States, 1990-1997: Results of a Follow-Up National Survey. *JAMA* 280: 1569-1575.

3. Borkan, J., Neher, J.O., Anson, O., and Smoker, B. (1994). Referrals for Alternative Therapies. *Journal of Family Practice* 39: 545-550.

Chapter 2

General Web Sites

SEARCH ENGINES

The following search engines are popular with librarians, students, and consumers. Most people need to quickly find basic information from a few good Web sites. They do not need pages and pages of every CAM Web site that exists on the Net!

Achoo Healthcare Online
<http://www.achoo.com/main.asp>

Achoo, produced by a Canadian company, calls itself a "gateway to health care." See the section "Alternative Medicine." Achoo is a terrific resource for CAM and traditional health information. It offers news, databases, discussion groups, products, and companies. Achoo gears its information toward both consumers and health professionals. Note that it features a very thorough segment for "newbies" (inexperienced Internet users) explaining all about search engines. Achoo includes "communities" that focus on topics such as women's health. The site is commercial, though, with numerous advertisements.

Dogpile
<http://www.dogpile.com>

Claiming "All results, no mess," Dogpile began in 1996 and is now owned and operated by InfoSpace, Inc., a wireless and

Internet solutions company marketing its services to businesses. Dogpile is a meta-search engine: it searches several search engines simultaneously (About, Ask Jeeves, Google, and more). It claims to give more comprehensive and relevant search results. Dogpile is commercial, accepting advertisements. Search by specific keywords and click the "fetch" button, or go to "Web Directory" and select "Health," then "Alternative Medicine" and choose from the links that appear. The site highlights resources they have reviewed. Dogpile is a great jumping off point to some of the more unusual CAM therapies. Some categories featured include guides and advice, directories, conditions and illnesses, Eastern medicine, herbs, spirituality and the New Age movement, mind therapies, and news and articles. Be aware that some of the "featured listings" are commercial sites selling products.

Google
<http://www.google.com>

Select "Directory," then "Health," and then "Alternative" to see an elaborate listing of categories with the number of associated "hits" (Web pages found). Google ranks Web sites by how frequently sites link to them and integrates the resources from several smaller search engines. Medical school and public librarians love this search engine because it can quickly find biomedical sites to answer most reference questions asked during their shifts at the library reference desk. Google has provided me with the facts I need most of the time. Our hospital doctors love it, too! It is easy to find Usenet discussion groups (forums): click on the "Groups" tab and type in a word or phrase.

Health on the Net (HON) Foundation
<http://www.hon.ch/MedHunt>

HON is a nonprofit medical information gateway. Produced by Health on the Net Foundation in Switzerland, it is a highly respected site. HON began in 1995 when a meeting of sixty international telemedicine experts convened to discuss the use of the Internet in health care. The group, including officials from the National Library of Medicine and Dr. Michael DeBakey, voted to "create a permanent body that would . . . promote the effective and reliable use of the new technologies for telemedicine in healthcare around the world." Today HON works closely with the Swiss Institute of Bioinformatics and the University Hospitals of Geneva. HON (see Figure 2.1) includes the search engines MedHunt and HONselect. This is a fine resource to lead you to the most reliable Web sites. HON does the quality filtering for you. Look for their seal of approval. See "Web Sources for Alternative Medicine." Visitors can search by language or topic.

Mamma
<http://www.mamma.com>

Mamma was created in 1996 as a student's master's thesis. Mamma is now owned by Intasys Corporation. The site is called the "mother of all search engines." Mamma (see Figure 2.2) sifts through several search engines simultaneously (meta-search engine). It is a good place to look for obscure (hard-to-find, unusual, rare, or new) topics. Select "Web," "News," "Images," etc. Type in a word or phrase and click on the "Go Mamma" button. Note that you can also search "Pay As You Go" commercial sites. Advertised Web sites are featured under a "Mamma Recommends" heading. After Google, Mamma is my favorite search engine to unearth the Web sites with the hard-to-find information I need.

Yahoo
<http://www.yahoo.com>

Yahoo stands for "Yet Another Hierarchical Officious Oracle." Today it is produced by Yahoo! Inc. It was created in 1994

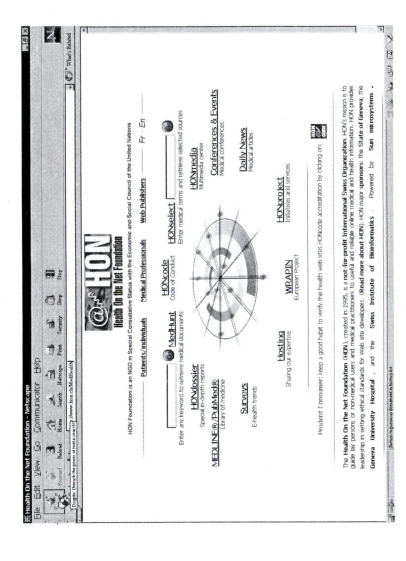

FIGURE 2.1. Health on the Net (HON) Foundation Home Page

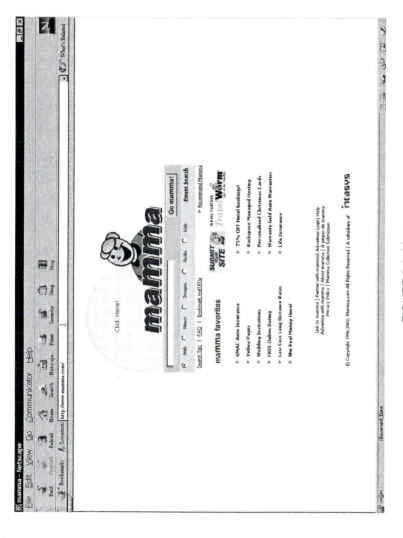

FIGURE 2.2. Mamma

17

by two Stanford University electrical engineering students. They first called it "Jerry's Guide to the World Wide Web." For CAM information, see the section "Yahoo Health, Alternative Medicine." Click on "Health" in the Web site directory, then select "Alternative Medicine." Yahoo is one of the most comprehensive search engines. Look at Q&As and the evaluations of therapies by well-known physicians (Nancy Snyderman and Andrew Weil). The featured Web sites are often suggested by users.

DISCUSSION GROUPS
(MAILING LISTS, CHAT ROOMS, NEWSGROUPS)

Good health and good sense are two of life's greatest blessings.

Publius Syrus, 42 B.C.

For detailed information on how to distinguish a mailing list (moderated and unmoderated) from a newsgroup, Usenet group, chat room, forum, online support group, or bulletin board, check out **Google Groups—Basics of Usenet** (http://groups. google.com/googlegroups/basics.html) or the explanations and links to other explanations on **Mossresourcenet** (http://www. mossresourcenet.org).

Generally, you "subscribe" or register to send and receive messages on a mailing list, online support group, or forum. Sometimes a "list owner" or moderator sets ground rules for participating in discussions and posting messages. Some groups are "chatty" and generate dozens of messages each day. With most chat rooms, bulletin boards, and Usenet groups, there is no need to subscribe. You simply access the group's Internet site and scan current and archived messages and decide whether you want to join in the message threads. *Warning:* Messages may be saved (archived) for public access or access by group members, so do not divulge personal information or write anything you would be embarrassed for outsiders to read. See the section Netiquette (Chapter 1) for more advice.

Another word of caution: It is difficult to verify the credentials (background, authority, honesty, knowledge) of discussion group participants. Never act on any advice offered by participants without checking first with your health care provider (even if the person in the chat room says he or she is a physician or "expert"). Be careful!

Google Groups
<http://www.google.com>

This is a segment on the main Google.com site. Click on the tab "Groups," and then type a word or phrase. Google Groups lists Usenet (newsgroups) discussion forums. Search the keyword "complementary" and choose your topic of interest from the postings. The site has an excellent FAQs section which answers beginner's questions about searching and using newsgroups.

Onelist.com (see Yahoo! Groups)

Self-Help Group Sourcebook Online
<http://www.mentalhelp.net/selfhelp>

The Self-Help Group Sourcebook is published by Mental Help Net. This is a fine place to look for information on online support groups. It is international in scope. Users can search by keywords. The information is provided by the Behavioral Health Center of St. Clare's Health Services in Denville, New Jersey. Note that you are connected to the names of actual support groups, not online forums.

SupportPath.com
<http://www.supportpath.com>

SupportPath.com provides links to support-related online chat rooms, bulletin boards, local and national support organizations, and information on dozens of health and relationship subjects. It was formerly called Support-Group.com. Support-Path's philosophy is that the opportunity to participate in Internet discussion groups gives people information, an opportunity to share experiences (and not feel alone), a chance to vent emotions, and a feeling of hope. Participants display artwork and poetry, and share personal stories.

Topica
<http://www.liszt.com>

Select "Health and Fitness" and then choose "Alternative Medicine." Topica gives specific instructions on subscribing to a particular mailing list. For example, do you need the approval of the mailing list moderator in order to subscribe? Topica includes the following information for each mailing list: list name, purpose, type (moderated or unmoderated), archive access (past postings), date mailing list was created, owner, and statistics (number of subscribers, average number of messages per day [chattiness factor]).

Topica also has a category for support groups which may be useful for CAM information. With Topica, you can also start your own mailing list. "Topica Exchange" allows you to start and manage your own e-mail discussion list or e-mail newsletter. Registration is required. See "Free List Hosting." Topica also offers commercial e-mail newsletter publishing services.

Yahoo! Groups (formerly **Onelist.com**)
<http://groups.yahoo.com>

This is part of Yahoo.com. You can create your own discussion group here (free, easy instructions, but registration is
required). To browse CAM groups, select "Health and Wellness," then "Alternative Medicine," and then browse specialized
groups for specific therapies.

MEGASITES (MEDICAL SCHOOL, ACADEMIC, OR LIBRARY BASED)

Knowledge itself is power.

Sir Francis Bacon (1561-1626)

These sites were selected from a large group of excellent resources. This is not an exhaustive listing. You may want to
check your local medical school, hospital, and public library
Web sites for additional useful CAM links.

The Alternative Medicine HomePage
<http://www.pitt.edu/~cbw/altm.html>

The Alternative Medicine HomePage is the winner of several
medical and wellness Internet awards. This well-organized, unbiased site is also one of the most comprehensive and up-to-date
sites. It is maintained by University of Pittsburgh librarian
Charles Wessel, who is an authority on CAM Internet resources;
he leads workshops teaching other medical librarians about
CAM resources on the Internet. Wessel gives one of the most
thorough definitions of CAM and clearly explains the differ-
ences between alternative and complementary medicine. The
Web site is divided into the following areas: "AIDS and HIV,"

"Internet Resources," "Mailing Lists and Newsgroups," "Government Resources," "Pennsylvania Resources," "Practitioners Directories," and "Related Resources." You could begin and end your search for CAM resources with this site. Bookmark it!

Bastyr University Library
<http://www.bastyr.edu>

Bastyr University in Seattle, Washington, educates CAM practitioners, provides clinical services, and conducts research in the area of natural health sciences (naturopathic medicine). It is interesting to see the high educational requirements for would-be naturopathic practitioners who choose to receive their education at Bastyr University. The school has been in existence for over twenty-five years. The Web site is arranged like that of traditional university Web sites, with an index on the left side and links to the library, news, and events on the right side. Note the special section for the general public. Rather unusual, though, is the "Recipe of the Month." Visitors can sign up to receive Bastyr University's free e-mail newsletter.

CAMPS (Complementary and Alternative Medicine Program at Stanford)
<http://camps.stanford.edu>

The purpose of CAMPS is "to study the effects of [CAM] therapies that may enhance successful aging . . . especially those therapies that may decrease the impact of cardiovascular and musculoskeletal diseases." CAMPS is based at the Stanford Center for Research in Disease Prevention, part of the Stanford University School of Medicine in Palo Alto, California. This is an example of how traditional medical education institutions in the United States have embraced the tenets of CAM.

Complementary and Alternative Medicine—Arizona Health Sciences Library
<http://www.ahsl.arizona.edu/>

Select "Web Links," then "Alternative Medicine." Librarians select the listed sites that, generally, are peer reviewed and do not rely heavily on advertising. The site is maintained by librarian Cathy Wolfson and is a basic yet thorough reference resource. Simply arranged, it consists of an alphabetical listing of recommended CAM sites, with links and a short description.

Complementary and Alternative Medicine—OHSU Holistic Medicine Interest Group
<http://www.ohsu.edu/ohmig/cam.html>

OHSU is the Oregon Health and Science University in Portland. The Web site includes brief summaries of included Internet links and useful sections on online journals and newsletters. This is another plain academic site, but it is easy to navigate with categories such as "Academic Institutions," "General Links," "Journals," "Organizations," "Specific Therapies," and "Student Resources." The Web site has not been updated in three years, but most of the links function.

HealthyNJ: Information for Healthy Living
<http://www.healthynj.org/>

HealthyNJ provides well-balanced information, including links to recommended Web sites, descriptions, newsgroups, and online support. The site was created by several librarians serving on the Consumer Health Information Task Force and is sponsored by The University of Medicine and Dentistry of New Jersey. Select the tab for "Health and Wellness" and then browse the alphabetical list of topics. Some listings are bilingual (Spanish). Many New Jersey resources are available.

McMaster University's Alternative Medicine Health Care Information Resources
<http://hsl.mcmaster.ca/tomflem/altmed.html>

This Canadian resource includes a link to an online dictionary, the *Expanded Dictionary of Metaphysical Healthcare.* The resources are aimed at health professionals as well as patients and their families. The site clearly indicates when it was last updated. Sites marked with a Canadian flag have a Canadian orientation. Be sure to look at CAMline (evidence-based CAM) and the Canadian Complementary Medical Association. There are general as well as specific CAM therapy sites. It is international in scope. McMaster University is a leader in providing information on evidence-based (research-proven) treatment, both traditional and CAM. Tom Flemming, a health sciences librarian, created and maintains the site.

MedWeb
<http://www.medweb.emory.edu/MedWeb/>

This is a comprehensive site maintained by the staff of the Woodruff Health Sciences Center Library of Emory University in Atlanta, Georgia. It is a bare bones Web site but very easy to navigate. Choose "Search All Subjects," then select "Alternative and Complementary Medicine" or "Focus Further."

MEL: Alternative Medicine/Unconventional Therapy
<http://mel.lib.mi.us/health/health-alternative.html>

Michigan Electronic Library (MEL) is the state library Web site for Michigan. This site is very well organized and easy to navigate (as would be expected from a Web site designed by librarians). Librarians tend to see questions (CAM and traditional medical) both in terms of the person asking the question (library "clients") and the person trying to find the answer for the client (the librarian). The Web sites designed by librarians tend to be clear and full of useful information. There is no razzle dazzle, just the facts. The Web site developers explain that they include some commercial sites for their informational value, basically the same reason I include such resources in this book. MEL includes links to specific therapies as well as general sites covering links to organizations and government and academic CAM sites. The specific therapy links are in a yellow box on the right. Other links are on the left ("Government Information Suppliers," "Academic Information Suppliers," "Associations," and "Additional Sources of Information").

NOAH: Alternative (Complementary) Medicine
<http://www.noah-health.org>

New York Online Access to Health (NOAH) is a real winner, very colorful and attractively arranged. Updated sites are identified, and new additions are clearly marked. This site is easy to navigate and it is fully bilingual (Spanish). NOAH is a collaborative effort between public and medical librarians, which probably accounts for its high quality. It provides a wealth of information on CAM, as well as traditional medicine. Just click on "Health Topics," then select "Complementary and Alternative Medicine." You can also browse the subject index or do a keyword search. Subtopics are arranged into "The Basics," "Resources," "Conditions," and "Anatomy." The site lists support groups. Be sure to read the sections "Fraud" and "Online Journals." NOAH (see Figure 2.3) is a top pick on many lists for general consumer health information, too.

Rosenthal Center for Complementary and Alternative Medicine
<http://www.rosenthal.hs.columbia.edu/>

One of the Rosenthal Center's objectives is to facilitate and conduct rigorous scientific investigation to evaluate the effec-

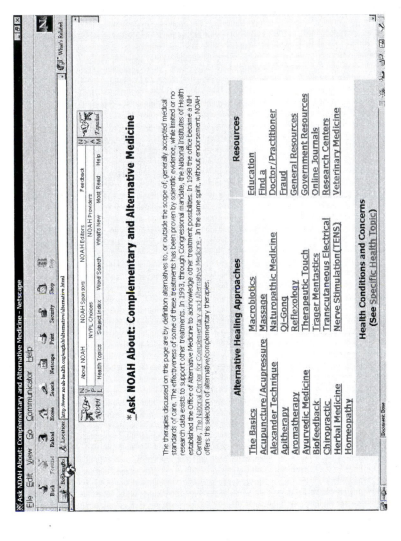

FIGURE 2.3. NOAH Complementary and Alternative Medicine Page

26

tiveness, safety, and mechanisms of action of CAM remedies and practice. The center (see Figure 2.4) aims to serve as a resource for its broad range of patients, is affiliated with Columbia University in New York City, and was one of the first CAM centers based at a medical school. The site is very attractive and easy to navigate. The Center has strong educational and research initiatives. It aims to educate both the public and health professionals. Select "CAM Research and Information Resources." Look at the Carol Ann Schwartz Cancer Education Initiative and explore "Carol Ann's Library," which provides information on CAM and pediatric cancers.

ASSOCIATIONS/ORGANIZATIONS

Included here are Web sites of several disease-specific organizations that sponsor online support groups (where people may discuss CAM as well as traditional therapies) or contain sections on CAM. Additional disease and symptom sites are listed in Chapter 4. There are also some general CAM organization sites in this section, but many additional association/organization sites exist. Consider using one of the search engines to find the Web sites of major diseases (especially chronic diseases). It may be helpful to think of organizations with major fund-raising drives (muscular dystrophy, breast cancer, and heart disease). These resources may emphasize traditional treatments, but many now include sections on CAM. It is important to be familiar with both types of treatment options.

Alternative Medicine Foundation, Inc.
<http://www.amfoundation.org>

The foundation is a nonprofit organization that produces the HerbMed and TibetMed databases (see Figure 2.5). Its mission is to provide evidence-based research resources for health care professionals and responsible, reliable information for patients

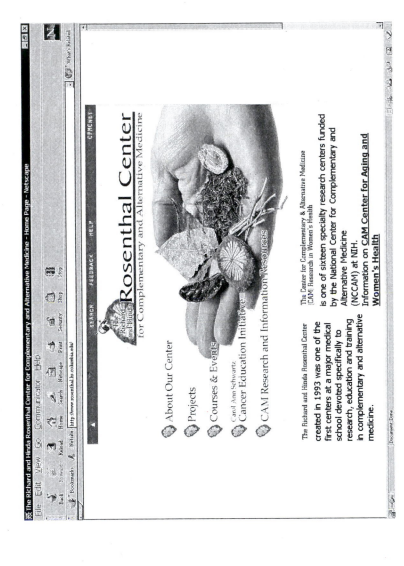

FIGURE 2.4. Rosenthal Center for Complementary and Alternative Medicine Home Page

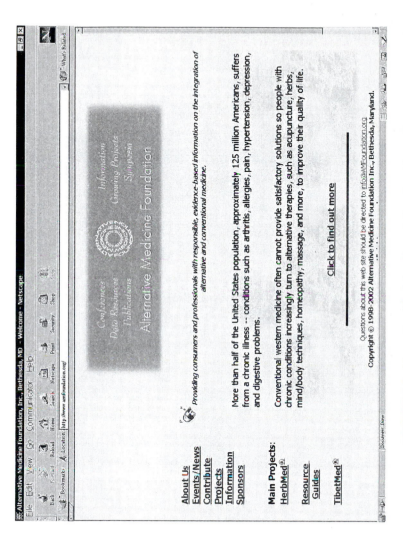

FIGURE 2.5. Alternative Medicine Foundation, Inc. Home Page

and consumers. The foundation tries to "conserve and respect the knowledge and practice of indigenous therapies and systems of healthcare." Part of its mission is to blend modern science with the promotion of health. Note the excellent resource guides to a dozen broad therapies. For anyone curious about the training a practitioner needs or seeking lists of recommended readings on a particular therapy, this is the site to examine. The HerbMed database allows visitors to search by keyword for references and research on the use of herbs to treat various illnesses. The HerbMed database includes adverse effects and categorizes the type of evidence that indicates how effective an herb is for treating a particular disorder. Physicians consult this database because it is one of the few CAM sites to examine the "evidence" (mainly rigorous research studies) with regard to the effectiveness of a CAM therapy. Select from the "Herb List" or type in the name of an herb. TibetMed has a library of questions and answers dealing with Tibetan medicine, but the site no longer accepts new questions. An international advisory board collaborated to create the Q&A library. The foundation offers a fee-based service, AskMed, developed with a physician who is board certified in family medicine. The physician answers brief questions and conducts telephone consultations for a fee.

American Cancer Society
<http://www.cancer.org>

The American Cancer Society is based in Atlanta, Georgia, with over 3,400 local offices. It is dedicated to the prevention of cancer, saving lives, and easing patients' suffering. The voluntary organization supports education, research, advocacy, and services. Parts of the Web site are available in Spanish (click on "Información en español"). Select the section "Patients, Family, and Friends" or "Choose a Cancer Type." Select "Search" and type in "alternative" to bring up dozens of links. View the table of contents of the *American Cancer Society Complementary and Alternative Cancer Methods Handbook* or read the society's guidelines for using dietary supplements and other CAM therapies. The section "Discussion" includes message boards and moderated (someone in authority leads the discussions or monitors the chats) live chat. It is necessary to register to join the online communities, but registration is free.

American Council for Headache Education (ACHE) <http://www.achenet.org>

ACHE was created in 1990 by the American Headache Society, an organization of 2,400 health professionals. ACHE's mission is to reach patients, their families, and employers. Much misunderstanding is related to chronic headaches and the people who suffer from headaches. See the section on nonpharmacological strategies for preventing migraine headaches, which details behavioral treatments (biofeedback, relaxation training, hypnosis, and stress-management training) and physical treatments (acupuncture, massage, manipulation of the cervical [neck] area). Select the "Art Museum" section to view drawings and paintings by headache sufferers. (See Figure 2.6.)

American Diabetes Association <http://www.diabetes.org>

The American Diabetes Association is a national nonprofit organization providing the public and health professionals with information and advocacy; it also supports research. Choose "Community and Resources" and then "Community Forums" for the opportunity to "share your ideas and opinions on a variety of topics with people affected with diabetes." The "Healthy Living" section offers nutritional guidance as well as tips on reducing stress.

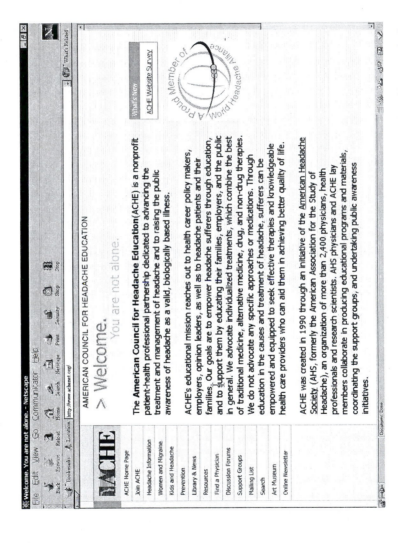

FIGURE 2.6. American Council for Headache Education Home Page. Reprinted by permission of the American Council for Headache Education.

Arthritis Foundation
<http://www.arthritis.org>

The Arthritis Foundation is a national nonprofit group that supports education, research, services, and advocacy for arthritis and related diseases. The Web site is attractively designed. Choose from tabs across the top, such as "Communities" for message boards. Also see "Consult and Control," an eighteen-week online program that guides participants on a physical activity program with weekly personalized e-mails (users must first fill out a questionnaire). Other segments include "Conditions and Treatments," "Talk About It," and "Focus on You." The Web site covers topics such as exercise, nutrition, pain management, emotional support, treatment options, and management of stress and depression. The fibromyalgia self-help course covers wellness skills, including exercise. The site is also available in Spanish. Select "Español" at the top of the home page.

Association for Integrative Medicine
<http://www.integrativemedicine.org>

The emphasis is on health care professionals, providing a forum for their research and communications. The association develops standards of practice and professional credentialing. The board of directors includes physicians, PhDs, nurses, and physical therapists. The association believes that diverse therapies, such as yoga, massage, hypnosis, and biofeedback, can work in conjunction with Western medicine. According to the Web site, "This integrated approach ultimately will lead to safer, faster, and more effective healthcare." Another part of its mission is to educate the public. Read the section "Education" for definitions of "holism" and "holistic health." Scroll down to the middle of the home page and select "On-line Library."

Endometriosis Association/Endo-Online
<http://www.endometriosisassn.org>

The Endometriosis Association is a nonprofit, self-help group. It was founded by women for women and aims to educate both patients and health professionals. The association also promotes research. Click on "Treatment Options" on the left side of the home page, and then select "Alternative Treatment." Visitors can purchase books online. Check out Endo-Online to find out about live (telephone, not online) support groups and chapters. The site includes correspondence networks and informal "crisis call" help.

Leukemia and Lymphoma Society
<http://www.leukemia.org>

The Leukemia and Lymphoma Society is a national voluntary health organization. It funds research, patient services, education, and patient advocacy. The mission of the society is to fight blood-related cancers (leukemias, lymphomas, Hodgkin's disease, myelomas) and "to improve the quality of life of patients and their families." The site includes several discussion boards or forums: "Living with Uncertainty," "Insurance Issues," "Parenting Issues" ("When a Child Has Cancer"), "When a Parent Has Cancer," "Coping With Treatment," and "Open Forum" (miscellaneous topics). CAM issues can be discussed within any of these forums. *Note:* Registration is required to post new messages and reply to others' messages.

National Alliance for the Mentally Ill (NAMI)
<http://www.nami.org>

NAMI, a national nonprofit organization for support, self-help, and patient advocacy, calls itself "the nation's voice on mental illness." Click on "Consumer Outreach" and then select "Support" to find local affiliates for live (telephone or in-person) contacts. There are dozens of online fact sheets on illnesses and medications (some are written in Spanish).

Physicians Committee for Responsible Medicine (PCRM)
<http://www.pcrm.org>

PCRM describes itself as "doctors and laypersons working together for compassionate and effective medical practice, research, and health promotion." This resource has a very good section labeled "Health." It emphasizes preventive medicine and nutrition (especially vegetarian diets). There are recipes for low-fat, heart-healthy dishes. PCRM launched television ads warning of the dangers of high-protein, low-carbohydrate diets, and the PCRM Web site discusses medical research studies supporting their opinion. PCRM's Cancer Project produced and distributed booklets and fact sheets on foods that may prevent certain types of cancer. PCRM.org sells books on related topics, and the site links to the American Holistic Medical Association.

Planetree/Planetree Model
<http://www.planetree.org>

Planetree was founded in 1978. The Planetree Model (see Figure 2.7) of health care sees the patient as an individual with a desire for self-determination regarding his or her own care. Planetree's mission is holistic and integrates massage and mind-body therapies with traditional Western medicine. Aromatherapy, pet therapy, consumer health libraries, and innovative design of patient areas are frequently part of Planetree-affiliated hospitals. The Web site includes a listing of affiliated hospitals.

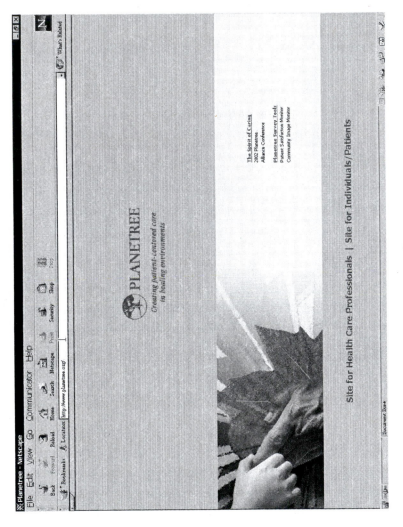

FIGURE 2.7. Planetree

The Wellness Community
<http://www.thewellnesscommunity.org>

The mission of the Wellness Community is to "help people with cancer fight for their recovery by providing free psychological and emotional support as an adjunct to conventional medical treatment." Wellness Communities exist in many cities across the United States, and they emphasize positive attitudes, stress management, proper nutrition, and participation in support groups. The site includes the personal stories of some participants, including physicians; these personal narratives are very inspirational. Join online support groups (click on the link on the left side of the home page) to link to the "Virtual Wellness Community." There are weekly and monthly online support groups providing educational and emotional support.

GENERAL CAM WEB SITES (NOT PRODUCED BY LIBRARIES, UNIVERSITIES, OR MEDICAL SCHOOLS)

This is a sampling of general CAM resources on the Internet. *Warning:* The credibility gets a bit muddied, even with those listed here, because so many have commercial links. Most of these sites sell books, films, tapes, vitamins, supplements, or services. I included these resources because they have value in their other features.

Alternative Medicine Center (HealthWorld Online)
<http://www.healthy.net/clinic/therapy/index.html>

The Alternative Medicine Center's advisory board includes an impressive group of MDs, DOs, PhDs, herbalists, acupuncturists, and a holistic nurse. The site (see Figure 2.8) aims to

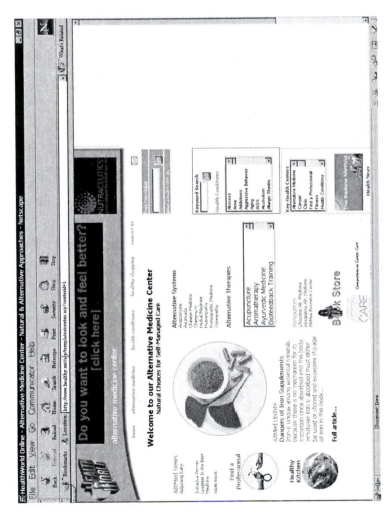

FIGURE 2.8. Alternative Medicine Center Home Page. Reprinted by permission of the Alternative Medicine Center of HealthWorld Online (www.healthy.net).

provide "natural choices for self-managed care." The Alternative Medicine Center is easy to browse. Do a keyword search or select sections such as "Alternative Medicine News," "Alternative Medicine Update," "Alternative Systems," "Alternative Therapies," and "Bookstore." Browse the listings under "Health Conditions." The Alternative Medicine Center features articles on both alternative and conventional treatments for common conditions. Read featured news stories and updates. Health-World Online, Inc., the parent Web site of the Alternative Medicine Center, is a commercial Web site selling a variety of products. It is a Los Angeles-based Internet health network integrating "both alternative and conventional health information into a synergistic whole."

Alternatives for Healthy Living
<http://www.alt-med-ed.com>

This Web site includes clear, lengthy descriptions and histories of many CAM therapies, lists conditions that may be treated by means of specific CAM therapies, and includes a list of organizations to contact. Note the names of dozens of CAM forums (moderated discussion groups) arranged by specific topic (for example, "Acupuncture Forum," "Color Therapy Forum," "Art Therapy Forum"). Click on the tabs for "Chat Rooms," "Advisories and Warnings," and "Keyword Search." The "Main Forum" features discussions around broad categories such as "Healthy Eating," "Weight Control," and "Anxiety."

Dr. Weil.com
<http://www.drweil.com>

The site is produced by Polaris Health, a holding company founded and controlled by Dr. Andrew Weil. The site is fairly commercial, but Dr. Weil's professional credentials are excellent (AB degree in biology [botany], MD degree, professor of internal medicine, and founder and director of the Program in Integrative Medicine at the University of Arizona Health Sciences Center). His books are in most public libraries, and he frequently appears on national public television. Dr. Weil defines integrative medicine as combining "the best ideas and practices of alternative and conventional medicine in order to maximize the body's natural healing mechanisms." His views on diet and nutrition are not extreme or overly restrictive. To navigate the site, select tabs such as "Discussions," "Ask Dr. Weil," and "Balanced Living."

Healthyroads
<http://www.healthyroads.com>

This Web site dubs itself "your online partner for wellness and health." The aim of Healthyroads is to help consumers educate themselves about CAM options for treating chronic medical conditions, with an emphasis on dietary supplements. The site sells tapes, books, vitamins, and dietary supplements; has a useful interaction guide to dietary supplements; and includes over 1,000 peer-reviewed articles on CAM. A wide variety of practitioners are on its editorial board (dentists, physicians, nurses, dietitians, and physical therapists).

Natural Health Center
<http://www2.womens-health.com/>

Natural Health Center is part of Women's Health Interactive. Choose "Health Centers" and then "Natural Health Center." The intent of the site is to empower "women through knowledge and action." It sees natural therapy as being one of three types: herbal medicine, homeopathy, or nutritional supplementation. Select "Resources" to link to electronic newsletters, support groups, and organizations. "Virtual Health for Women" is a free biweekly electronic newsletter. The tab "Discussion" brings up links to topic-specific discussion groups.

Natural Health Line
<http://www.naturalhealthvillage.com>

This resource is sponsored by Amazon.com, the online bookseller, and includes news and advice on how to find a naturopathic practitioner. The news links are current and cover hot topics reported on news wires such as Reuters, television networks, and national and international newspapers.

Rx List (The Internet Drug Index): Alternatives
<http://www.rxlist.com/alternative.htm>

The Web site is owned and operated by RxList, LLC. Neil Sandow, PharmD, a licensed pharmacist for over twenty years, founded and maintains RxList. A nifty search engine allows visitors to type in an alternative medication (try "feverfew") and request long or short documentation. RxList (see Figure 2.9) frequently warns of dangers or possible side effects, and the site advises consultation with one's doctor or pharmacist before taking any of the herbs or other substances. The site is both fun to use and informative. RxList gives less information than HerbMed, but it is fast and authoritative.

Yahoo! Guide to Alternative Medicine
<http://dir.yahoo.com//Health/Alternative_Medicine>

This is a gateway (portal) to products, therapies, and organizations. It categorizes Web sites according to popularity (sites that get the most "hits" on the Yahoo! search engine).

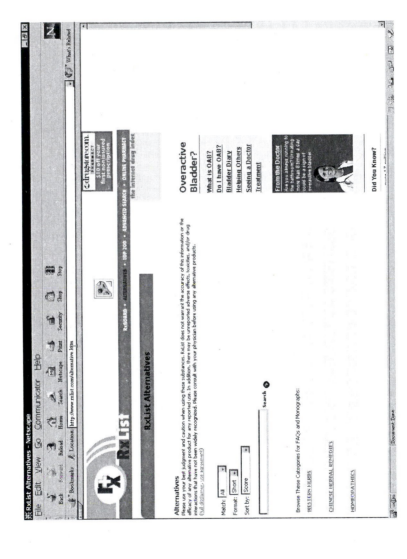

FIGURE 2.9. Rx List

GENERAL GOVERNMENT RESOURCES

This is a selection representing some of the best U.S. government CAM sites. Other countries, particularly Canada and Great Britain, also have excellent resources.

Healthfinder (Alternative Medicine)
<http://www.healthfinder.gov>

Healthfinder (see Figure 2.10) was developed by the U.S. Department of Health and Human Services and is excellent at pulling together quality information. It includes federal-government-sponsored publications, support/self-help groups, information clearinghouses, databases, and nonprofit organizations. Select "Alternative Medicine." It offers a free guide to reliable consumer health and human services information.

MEDLINEplus and MEDLINEplus Spanish Language
<http://www.medlineplus.gov>
<http://www.medlineplus. gov/esp>

MEDLINEplus is a service of the National Library of Medicine and the National Institutes of Health (see Figure 2.11). It offers one-stop shopping for health information for consumers and health professionals. MEDLINEplus includes links to major government and organization health sites, a medical dictionary, drawings, and the PubMed database of medical journal articles which can be searched by disease topics. Be sure to check out the PubMed CAM subset, which automatically limits articles to those on CAM. Public libraries can help to obtain copies of the articles referenced. Some medical school libraries are open to the public (usually during weekdays, sometimes for a fee) and may have coin-operated photocopiers for copying articles. You should call ahead first for access policies. A Spanish-language version is now available (www.medlineplus.gov/esp).

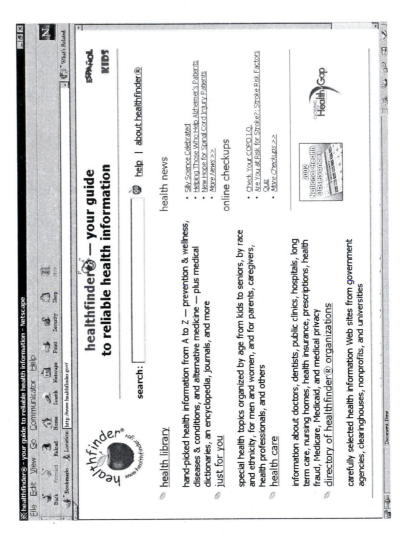

FIGURE 2.10. Healthfinder Home Page

44

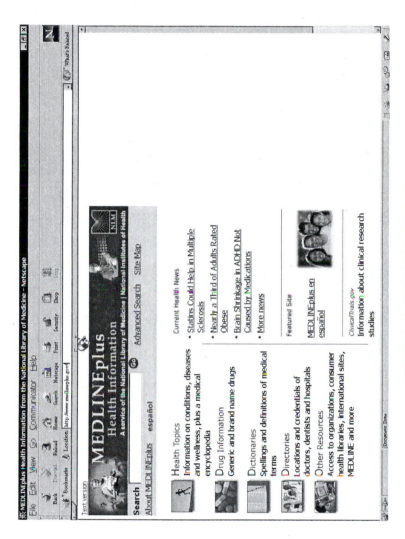

FIGURE 2.11. MEDLINEplus Home Page

This is one of the best consumer resources for reliable, unbiased CAM and traditional medical information. Public libraries in many cities are publicizing MEDLINEplus and making special efforts to teach the public how to use its features effectively, but the site is very user friendly. Click on the arrow on the left side for "Health Topics" and "Drug Directories." Check back frequently for new sections, drugs, and diseases.

National Center for Complementary and Alternative Medicine (NCCAM)
<http://nccam.nih.gov>

NCCAM (see Figure 2.12) was established to supervise a dozen Centers for CAM Research to evaluate alternative treatments for many chronic medical conditions and specialty areas (addictions, aging, arthritis, cancer, cancer and hyperbaric oxygenation, cardiovascular diseases, cardiovascular disease and aging in African Americans, chiropractic, craniofacial disorders, neurological disorders, neurodegenerative disorders, and pediatrics). NCCAM's mission is rigorous scientific evaluation of the most promising alternative medical practices. NCCAM defines alternative and complementary medicine as "those treatments and healthcare practices not taught widely in medical schools, not generally used in hospitals, and not generally reimbursed by medical insurance companies." See their online publication "Are You Considering Complementary and Alternative Medicine (CAM)?" To access this publication, select "Health Information" and then choose "Making Decisions About Using CAM."

The site covers topics to consider before selecting alternative therapy or an alternative treatment practitioner. There are online fact sheets on acupuncture, St. John's wort, and hepatitis C. The online newsletter *Complementary and Alternative Medicine at the NIH* can be accessed at this site. Note the segment "Alerts and Advisories" for information on ephedra, kava, and bioterrorism. Overall, this is one of the best online resources on CAM because

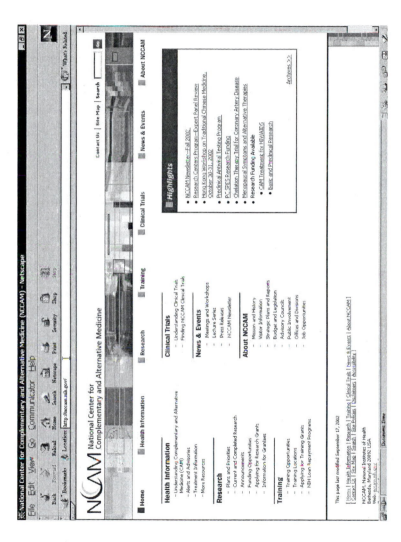

FIGURE 2.12. NCCAM Page

the centers try to present evidence that specific CAM treatments are effective.

The specialty centers, most with their own Web sites, are as follows:

- Center for Addiction and Alternative Medicine Research (Minnesota)
  <http://www.mmrfweb.org/research/addiction&alt_med/index.html>
- Center for CAM Research in Aging and Women's Health (New York)
  <http://cpmcnet.columbia.edu/dept/rosenthal>
- Center for Alternative Medicine Research on Arthritis (Maryland)
  <http://www.compmed.ummc.umaryland.edu>
- Center for Cancer Complementary Medicine (Maryland)
  <http://www.hopkins-cam.org>
- Specialized Center of Research in Hyperbaric Oxygen Therapy (Pennsylvania)
- CAM Research Center for Cardiovascular Diseases (Michigan)
  <http://www.med.umich.edu/camrc/index.html>
- Center for Natural Medicine and Prevention (Iowa)
  <http://mum.edu/CNMP>
- Consortial Center for Chiropractic Research (Iowa)
  <http://www.palmer.edu>
- Oregon Center for Complementary and Alternative Medicine Research in Craniofacial Disorders (Oregon)
- Oregon Center for Complementary and Alternative Medicine in Neurological Disorders (Oregon)
- Center for CAM in Neurodegenerative Diseases (Georgia)
  <http://www.emory.edu/WHSC/MED/Neurology/CAM/index.html>
- Pediatric Center for Complementary and Alternative Medicine (Arizona)

National Diabetes Information Clearinghouse: Alternative Therapies for Diabetes
<http://www.niddk.nih.gov>

This Web site covers acupuncture, biofeedback, dietary supplements (chromium, magnesium, vanadium), and guided imagery to aid in the treatment of diabetes and its many severe complications. Because diabetes and its complications can be life threatening, patients should be especially careful to work closely with their physician or nurse practitioner. This is the only site on CAM and diabetes that I consider prudent in its advice to diabetics. Select "Diabetes" under "Health Information," then "Alternative Therapies for Diabetes" under "Diabetes Topics." In this segment read about the use of acupuncture, biofeedback, and several dietary supplements.

Office of Cancer Complementary and Alternative Medicine (OCCAM)
<http://www3.cancer.gov/occam>

OCCAM (see Figure 2.13) conducts research and provides information for consumers and health practitioners on CAM therapies for cancer. Like the other government CAM resources, OCCAM researches the evidence that particular treatments are effective. OCCAM has a clean, well-arranged design. The right side of the home page features "News," "Workshops," "Research," and "Alerts and Advisories."

U. S. Food and Drug Administration
<http://www.fda.gov>

(See Herbal Medicine section in Chapter 3.)

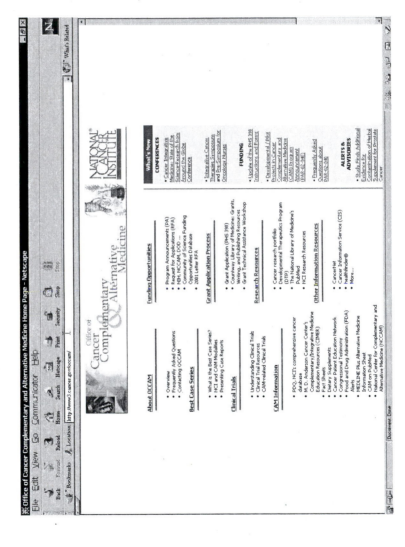

FIGURE 2.13. OCCAM Home Page

50

White House Commission on Complementary and Alternative Medicine Policy
\<http://whccamp.hhs.gov>

President Bill Clinton, through Executive Order 13147, authorized the creation of the commission on March 7, 2000. The full text of the commission's final report (March 2002) is accessible here. The commission is charged with researching CAM practices and products. Some additional charges are as follows:

- *Delivery of and public access to CAM services:* This involves dissemination of reliable information on CAM to health care providers and the general public.
- *Appropriate licensing, education, and training of CAM health care practitioners:* The commission's recommendations on public policy and legislation went to President George W. Bush (via the Secretary of Health and Human Services) in 2002. The transcripts of the commission's meetings are available here.

Chapter 3

A Sampling of CAM Therapies
and Philosophies

Included in this chapter are a few of the most popular CAM treatments and fields of knowledge. This is not meant to be an exhaustive listing of all treatments or all Web sites under each treatment category. I selected sites that are representative of their category or have particularly useful features or links to related sites. In general, I have tried to include no more than two or three sites per category. You should explore for yourself and try to find other Web sites which you enjoy using and which have features for your particular circumstances.

ACUPUNCTURE

Acupuncture is the traditional Chinese practice of puncturing the skin in precise locations with fine needles to cure disease or to relieve pain. It was developed more than 3,000 years ago and is based on Taoist philosophy. It aims to balance the energy meridians to allow the body to heal itself.

Acupuncture.com
<http://www.acupuncture.com>

This Web site goes beyond acupuncture to include other traditional Chinese therapies such as massage, Chinese herbal medicine, and qi gong. The site is aimed at three different audiences: consumers/patients, practitioners, and students of traditional Chinese therapies. Site patrons can subscribe to the free e-mail newsletter "Points," on Chinese traditional therapies and acupuncture. "Ask the Doctor" provides referrals to acupuncturists and accepts questions from the public. There is a "Frequently Asked Questions" segment. The "Store" sells videos, books, herbs, and acupuncture supplies for practitioners and consumers. "Recipes," some homey, some therapeutic, are available online. The "Reference Library" is the most useful section, with full-text information on Chinese traditional therapies graded by level (consumer, student, or practitioner).

American Academy of Medical Acupuncture (AAMA)
<http://www.medicalacupuncture.org>

This Los Angeles-based organization is the sole physician-only professional acupuncture society in North America. Its purpose is to promote the integration of concepts from traditional and modern forms of acupuncture with Western medical training. When seeking an acupuncture practitioner, membership in this society should be part of the person's credentials. Click on "Find an Acupuncturist" and type in state or area code (not zip code) to see a list of AAMA-certified practitioners. Searching the "Public" area by medical condition keyword (try "migraine") brings up press releases, articles, and presentations on the application of acupuncture to ease the condition.

AFRICAN-AMERICAN WELLNESS

BlackHealthCare.com
<http://www.blackhealthcare.com>

This site (see Figure 3.1), directed by Arthur Beau White, PhD, deals with health issues of interest to people of color in the

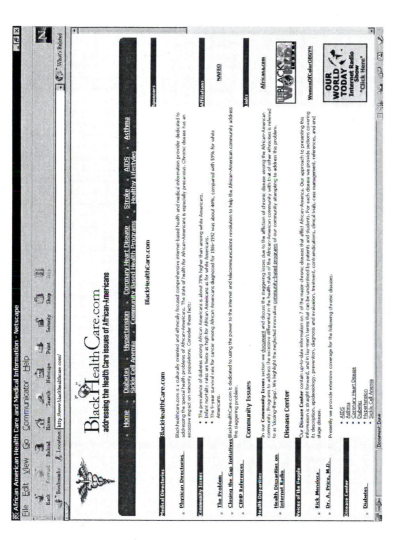

FIGURE 3.1. BlackHealthCare.com Home Page

55

United States. Topics of concern include chronic conditions such as diabetes, hypertension, asthma, and sickle-cell anemia. These disorders have a higher incidence in the African-American community. The information is presented in layman's terms, but it is based on material published in top medical journals. Although the site emphasizes traditional Western medicine, the site's producers plan to add information about traditional African herbal health remedies. BlackHealthCare.com also includes online discussion groups and sections on lifestyle issues such as finance and dating.

BlackWomensHealth.com
<http://www.blackwomenshealth.com>

"Dedicated to the health and wellness of today's African-American woman," this is a high-quality, authoritative site. It is produced by two physicians and was created in 1999 by David Pryor, MD, a specialist in internal medicine. See the excellent section "Dietary Supplements 101." The site's articles are written by health professionals, including nutritionists and physicians, with lists of references for further reading. To navigate BlackWomensHealth. com, click on tabs to links to discussions, a directory of physicians, events, and FAQs. See "BWH. com Community" for free registration to participate in forums moderated by a facilitator. "Chat Events" are planned for the future.

ALEXANDER TECHNIQUE (AT)

The Alexander technique (AT) was developed in the 1890s by F. M. Alexander, an Australian actor. Practitioners use gentle touch and observation to change the body's patterns of movement. A goal is reeducating the patient to change poor habits of coordination. Practitioners of the technique believe habits of excessive tension and inefficient coordination affect how one feels and thinks. The technique focuses on correct posture and the correct way to lift objects.

Alexander Technique
<http://www.life.uiuc.edu/jeff/alextech.html>

This Web resource includes names of some Alexander technique practitioners and provides links to a small number of sites on AT, AT teachers, societies, an online magazine, and a book publisher. The links to societies include detailed descriptions of the Alexander technique, articles, and notices of training workshops.

Alexander Technique International (ATI)
<http://www.ati-net.com>

ATI is a worldwide professional organization. This is a good place to look for listings of practitioners and places that offer training classes. The site includes the ATI certification standards and a code of ethics for teachers of the Alexander technique.

American Society for the Alexander Technique
<http://www.alexandertech.org>

This is the site of the largest professional association of board-certified Alexander technique teachers in the United States. The society offers courses leading to certification. The section "On-line Articles" includes a very thorough history of AT, an explanation of what occurs during a lesson, discussion of how the technique works, and how AT can be useful to people with chronic pain. Articles discuss AT's application for musicians, pregnant women, and computer users.

Complete Guide to the Alexander Technique
<http://www.alexandertechnique.com>

The Complete Guide was created by an AT teacher and author and his wife. It includes online articles about the use of AT training to ease or prevent various medical conditions, such as carpal tunnel syndrome and backache. The site explains what happens during a group lesson. There is a section on ergonomics. The guide thoroughly explains AT. See the segment "Alexander On-Line," a guide to interactive AT resources (bulletin boards, discussion groups, tutorials, "ask a question" services, etc.).

AROMATHERAPY

Aromatherapy is the topical or inhaled application of botanical oils (essential oils) extracted from barks, flowers, grasses, and herbs. Examples are lemon oil, sage, eucalyptus oil, and sandalwood. Aromatherapy is an ancient healing art that dates to 4,500 B.C.

AromaWeb
<http://www.aromaweb.com>

AromaWeb (see Figure 3.2) features recipes, book reviews, articles, and information on aromatherapy and the use of essential oils. It was created and is produced by Wendy Robbins, a professional Web site developer and designer. Select links on the left side of the home page or choose "Search AromaWeb" and type a keyword. Note the important section "Hazardous Essential Oil List" which appears in the "Oil Profiles" section. The list points out toxic oils that should be used only by qualified aromatherapy practitioners. Some oils should never be used for aromatherapy. Select "Recipe Box" for recipes in categories that include emotional well-being and physical well-

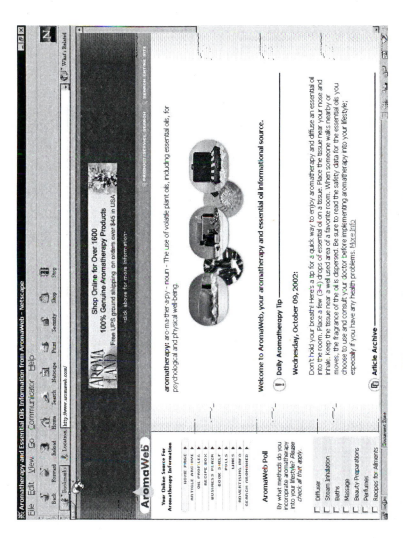

FIGURE 3.2. AromaWeb Home Page

being. The recipes are simple to follow. Note the four different anger-diffusing blends.

AYURVEDIC MEDICINE

This is the traditional Indian, nature-based health care aimed at achieving a state of balance between body and mind. Ayurveda offers multiple strategies for harmonizing mind, body, and spirit through herbs, diet, meditation, massage, aromatherapy, and self-healing regimens.

Ayurvedic and Siddha Medicine Internet Resources
<http://www.holisticmed.com/www/ayurvedic.html>

The Web site is produced by the Holistic Medicine Resource Center. It is very thorough and includes discussion groups, organizations, education, practitioners, and publications. *Note:* The site gives clear instructions on how to subscribe (sign up) to Internet discussion groups.

Ayurvedic Institute
<http://www.ayurveda.com>

The Ayurvedic Institute was established in 1984 "to teach and provide the traditional therapy of East Indian Ayurveda" and is located in Albuquerque, New Mexico. The Web site includes online articles about Ayurveda (see Figure 3.3). Read "Ayurveda: A Brief Introduction and Guide" by Dr. Vasant Lad for background information. Click on the lotus blossom buttons on the left side of the home page to access sections on "The Institute," "Education," and "Panchakarma." Panchakarma is a cleansing and rejuvenating program.

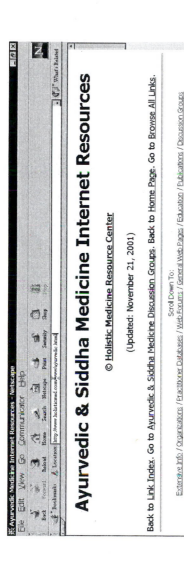

FIGURE 3.3. Ayurvedic and Siddha Medicine Internet Resources

BIOFEEDBACK

Biofeedback is sometimes called relaxation training or alpha control and is used to relieve pain, heal muscle injuries, relieve urinary (bladder) incontinence, and promote relaxation. It may involve placement of electrodes (sensors) on the head or other parts of the body to record the body's electrical patterns. The patient learns to control these electrical patterns by means of deep breathing and relaxation.

The Biofeedback Network (BN): Online Biofeedback Resources <http://www.biofeedback.net>

This is a commercial site, selling tapes, equipment, classified ads, and corporate programs. Biofeedback or relaxation training has been practiced by mainstream physicians and dentists for many years. Chronic pain conditions, such as headaches, often - respond to biofeedback. Click on the links to "Associations," "Biofeedback Centers," "Education," "Practitioners," "Equipment," "Marketplace," and "Events Calendar."

CHINESE OR ASIAN TRADITIONAL MEDICINE

American Association of Oriental Medicine (AAOM) <http://www.aaom.org>

AAOM (see Figure 3.4) is the umbrella organization representing the profession of acupuncture in the United States; it assisted in the formation of the National Commission for the Certification of Acupuncturists and the National Council of Acupuncture Schools and Colleges. The Web site has broadened its scope to include such areas as Chinese herbology, qi manipulation techniques, room arrangement, martial arts, and acupuncture. There is an excellent overview of Oriental medicine. Note

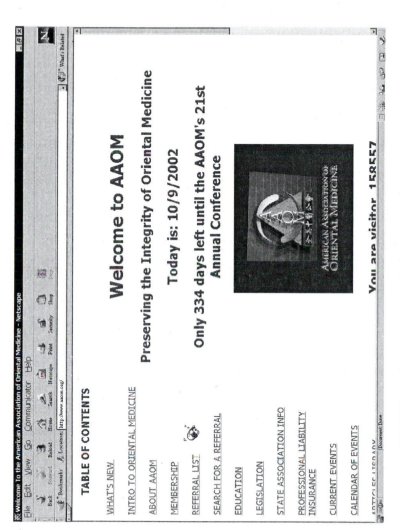

FIGURE 3.4. American Association of Oriental Medicine (AAOM)

the sections "How Acupuncture Works" and "How Acupuncture Feels." This Web site is a reliable resource for referral to certified acupuncturists.

Pro-Cultura's Web Site on Tibetan Medicine
<http://www.tibetmedicine.org>

This resource gives a very concise yet complete history of Tibetan medicine (see "What Is Tibetan Medicine?"). Pro-Cultura, Inc., is a nonprofit organization whose goal is to support collaboration between the biomedical (Western) sector and traditional (Eastern) health sector. Ultimately, the site's producers hope this collaboration will develop "sustainable solutions for improving global health equity." They aim to foster awareness of Tibetan medicine in North America. The site includes news, recommended reading, a list of Tibetan practitioners, and exhibitions.

TibetMed
<http://www.tibetmed.org>

TibetMed is maintained by the Alternative Medicine Foundation, Inc., a nonprofit organization that also produces the HerbMed Web site. TibetMed continues a dialogue begun in 1998 at the First International Congress on Tibetan Medicine in Washington, DC. Click on the link to the congress and read about the history of Tibetan medicine.

CHIROPRACTIC

This employs manipulation and adjustment of body structures (particularly the spine) to cure diseases through the restoration of normal nerve function. Chiropractic is commonly used to treat backache, chronic pain, and poor posture.

American Chiropractic Association (ACA)
<http://www.amerchiro.org>

ACA is the largest professional association of doctors of chiropractic medicine. As would be expected, the ACA covers the field very thoroughly (see Figure 3.5). It includes news on insurance coverage, consumer tips, a directory of doctors of chiropractic care, history of the profession, and frequently asked questions. Many major health insurers now cover chiropractic therapy, thanks in part to the ACA's lobbying efforts.

FELDENKRAIS WORK

Feldenkrais includes the principles developed by Moshe Feldenkrais and is based on physics and biomechanics. It employs gentle movement to gradually increase range of motion, flexibility, balance, and coordination. Feldenkrais attempts to reprogram the nervous system by means of movement supplemented by physical pressure and manipulation.

Feldenkrais Guild of North America
<http://www.feldenkrais.com>

The Web site of the Oregon-based guild provides information on finding Feldenkrais practitioners, training information, and general information about the Feldenkrais Method. The full name is the Feldenkrais Method of Somatic Education. This site discusses two variations: Functional Integration and Awareness Through Movement. Some hospitals offer Feldenkrais sessions (for a fee) to the public.

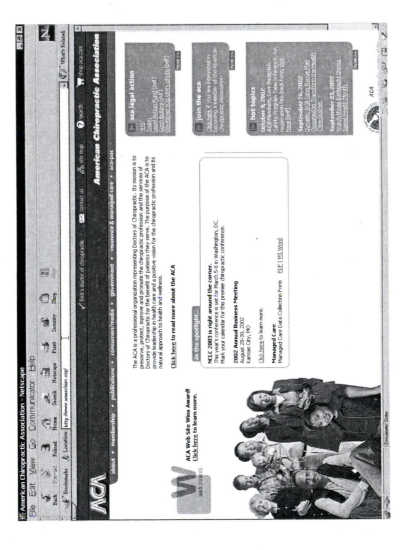

FIGURE 3.5. American Chiropractic Association Home Page

Feldenkrais Resources
<http://www.feldenkrais-resources.com>

The site lists workshops and classes, includes links to sites on other somatic methods (Rolfing, Alexander technique), and sells videos, tapes, and books (for example, Dr. Moshe Feldenkrais's books, including *Awareness Through Movement*). Note that the site also sells videos and texts on "Tellington Touch" (TTouch), the Feldenkrais method as applied to pets. See the Veterinary CAM section for the Tellington Touch Web site.

GUIDED IMAGERY (GI)

Guided imagery is the process of imaging through any of the senses (taste, touch, smell, hearing, and sight). Examples are biofeedback, hypnosis, desensitization, relaxation techniques, and transcendental meditation. GI often involves listening to music or a person's voice in a relaxed setting, so imagery and deep feelings can surface from one's inner self.

Academy for Guided Imagery Online
<http://www.interactiveimagery.com>

The mission of the academy is to use "the power of the mind for healing, growth, and creativity." The academy's program directors are a physician and a psychologist with extensive medical and CAM credentials. The academy educates and supports practicing clinicians in the use of imagery in therapy. The site includes a directory of practitioners of interactive guided imagery and also sells products for consumers who wish to use the self-healing tools to treat themselves. Click on links to learn about self-healing tools or to read about interactive guided imagery.

Guided Imagery
<http://www.guidedimageryinc.com>

Guided Imagery is commercial, but there is a good section on the application of guided imagery in health care. The site is produced by a registered nurse who is the former director of the Cleveland Clinic's Guided Imagery Program. She explains how to use the tapes and CDs sold on the site. The Web site is visually pleasing and simple to navigate. There is an informative section on stress and its symptoms.

HealthJourneys: Guided Imagery Resource Center
<http://www.guidedimagery.com>

This is a commercial site, selling tapes and CDs, but it has some worthwhile sections. There is an excellent explanation of the principles of guided imagery, and the section on tips for practicing guided imagery will be of great benefit to people who are new to the subject. Tapes are grouped by topics including weight loss, stress, cancer, heart health, and post-traumatic stress disorder. Click on links to "Research," "Interviews and Articles," and "Products." See "Give 'n Take" for the link to the discussion board "Talk Amongst Yourselves."

HERBAL MEDICINE

This is the practice of applying or administering specific herbs to treat medical problems.

American Botanical Council's *HerbalGram*
<http://www.herbalgram.org>

Some information on the site is accessible only to members (fee-based), but there are also free sections to browse. Read

HerbClip for news items. The American Botanical Council (ABC) is a nonprofit research and education organization. It educates the public by disseminating information based on scientific research. ABC promotes safe and effective use of herbs, including medical plants and phytomedicine.

Cyberbotanica: Plants and Cancer Treatments
<http://biotech.icmb.utexas.edu/botany/>

The site provides a "virtual chapter" on medicinal botany. Cyberbotanica is part of Indiana University's BioTech Project. The site provides information on botanical compounds used in cancer treatment and research, as well as the plants from which the compounds are extracted. The project is no longer funded, but the Internet links are kept up to date.

GRAS (Generally Recognized As Safe) List of Botanicals
<http://www.ars-grin.gov/duke/syllabus/gras.htm>

GRAS is a compilation of all botanicals appearing on the Food and Drug Administration's list of food additives generally recognized as safe by a consensus of scientific opinion. Read the introduction, which explains why some herbal products are safe, even though they might not appear on the GRAS list. GRAS is excerpted from the Code of Federal Regulations (CFR Title 21, Parts 172, 182, 184, and 186).

Henriette's Herbal Homepage
<http://www.ibiblio.org/herbmed/index.html>

Henriette Kress archives (stores) replies to the newsgroup alt.folklore.herbs, the Medicinal Herblist (a discussion group on medicinal and aromatic plants), and some other herbal discussion lists. The site provides information on culinary and medicinal herbs. Henriette has been dubbed the "herbal archivist of cyberspace." Read her "Medical Herb FAQ" and "Culinary FAQ." She selects the best of the herbal forums and organizes their archives by herb, problem, and other categories.

HerbMed
<http://www.herbmed.org>

HerbMed was developed by Soaring Bear, PhD, and is produced by Alternative Medicine Foundation, Inc. The site is an interactive electronic herbal database and provides access to scientific evidence-based data on the medicinal use of herbs. See the listing for the Alternative Medicine Foundation.

Herb Research Foundation
<http://www.herbs.org>

This is a nonprofit organization that publishes the *Herbal-Gram* newsletter. Membership (for a fee) provides access to various types of information; the fees vary by type of services provided. For additional information, see the section on the American Botanical Council's *HerbalGram*. Click on "Resources" for lists of schools, where to purchase herbs, reading lists, and practitioners. The "Bookstore" sells botanical and herb books. An "Ask the Experts" section posts answers to questions. Visitors can order, for a small fee, packets of information on specific conditions or herbs.

Herbal Medicine Center
<http://www.healthy.net>

This address brings visitors to HealthWorld Online. From here, select "Herbal Medicine" from the list on the left sidebar. This is the site of the Herbal Medicine Center. Sections include an introduction to herbs, herbs for specific conditions, herbs and women's health, herbs and men's health, herbs and children's health, and information on locating herbal practitioners.

Herbs and Aromas
<http://world.std.com/~krahe/>

This Web site provides information about medicinal plants and herbs. There are good definitions of terms such as tincture, decoction, syrup, infusion, cream, ointment, and essential oil. Select the "Do It Yourself" link on the home page to access detailed instructions for making oils and perfumes. There is information on how to dry and store herbs. Links include "In the Kitchen," "Herb Rings and Nets," "Alternative and Herbal Medicine," "Plant Images," and "Side Effects."

Howie Brounstein's Home
<http://home.teleport.com/~howieb/howie.html>

Howie Brounstein is the owner of Columbines and Wizardry Herbs, Inc.; he has taught botany, herbalism, and wildcrafting for twenty years. Currently, he offers intensive apprenticeship programs that include field trips and lectures. His home page includes a variety of herbal and botanical links, recipes for making herbal cough syrup, and information on using herbs to treat toothaches and minor cuts. To navigate the site, scroll down the page and click links of interest.

Mrs. Grieve's *A Modern Herbal*
<http://www.botanical.com>

This is a link on the Botanical.com Web site. Click on "Open and Read *A Modern Herbal*." The site includes medicinal, culinary, and cosmetic herbs. It was first published (in print format) in the 1930s. The site includes a message board and links to a company from which to purchase herbs. Choose "Plant and Herb Index," "Index of Recipes," and "Index of Poisons." Some of the listed herbs may be ordered online.

Native American Ethnobotany Database
<http://www.umd.umich.edu/cgi-bin/herb/>

The Native American Ethnobotany Database was created and is still produced by Dan Moerman, PhD, a professor of anthropology at the University of Michigan-Dearborn. He has been working on the project for over twenty-five years. The site (see Figure 3.6) includes foods, drugs, dyes, and fibers of the Native North American peoples. Type in keywords (try "headaches") and retrieve articles.

NIH's Office of Dietary Supplements: International Bibliographic Information on Dietary Supplements (IBIDS) Database of Dietary Supplement Literature
<http://ods.od.nih.gov/>

The Office of Dietary Supplements' mission is to strengthen knowledge and understanding of dietary supplements by disseminating results of research, educating the public, and evaluating scientific information to foster enhanced quality of life. I would check this resource and that of the U.S. Food and Drug Administration before considering the use of any supplements. See the section "Health Information" for dietary supplement fact sheets, safety notices, and the IBIDS consumer database. Try out the database by typing in "taurine," a supplement recommended on some low-carbohydrate diets as an alternative to diuretic medications.

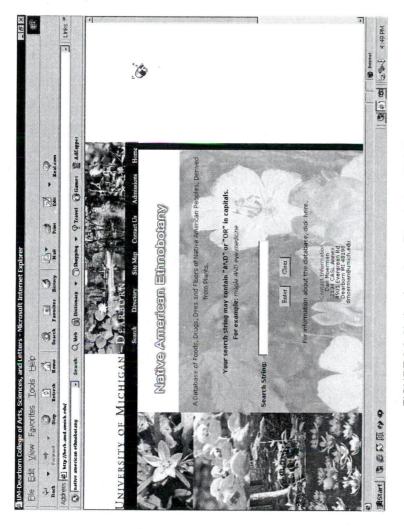

FIGURE 3.6. Native American Ethnobotany Database

Soaring Bear's Medicinal Herb Science Information
<http://Soaringbear.tripod.com>

"Medicinal Herb Science Information" is a section on Soaring Bear's (PhD in pharmacology) personal Web page. He is currently on staff at the National Library of Medicine. His links (references) are very useful for those who want to delve deeply into Native American traditional therapies. Read the information on sweat lodges, an ancient Native American body purification ceremony involving use of intense heat, similar to that of a sauna, to provoke insights and visions. Also, see the previous section on HerbMed, which was developed by Soaring Bear. The Web site is currently being redesigned.

Southwest School of Botanical Medicine (SSBM)
<http://www.all-natural.com/herbindx.html>

Michael Moore is the director of SSBM in Arizona. This is the place to look for images and video clips of medicinal plants (click on "Medicinal Plant Images"). The Web site also provides information about courses and various *materia medica* resources.

University of Washington's Medicinal Herb Garden
<http://nnlm.gov/pnr/uwmhg/index.html>

This is an actual herb garden located on the campus of the University of Washington in Seattle. Search plants by common or botanical name. Take a virtual tour (select "Walk Through the Garden"). The site was part of a demonstration project funded by the National Network of Libraries of Medicine, Pacific Northwest Region.

U.S. Food and Drug Administration
<http://www.fda.gov>

The FDA's mission is to promote and protect public health by helping safe and effective medical products reach the market in a timely way and monitoring products for continued safety after they are in use (see Figure 3.7). It would be wise to regularly check the section "Dietary Supplements" to see warnings regarding adverse effects. Read the "FDA News" and "Hot Topics" sections for current, vital information. Note the advice on buying medicines online, safety alerts, and warnings about ephedra.

HISPANIC HERBALISM

California School of Traditional Hispanic Herbalism
<http://www.HispanicHerbs.com>

This site does not provide specific herbal remedy recommendations. It focuses on offering online and on-site courses on *curanderismo* (native Hispanic California healing philosophies and techniques). Clicking on the links to the online classes will provide brief descriptions of what constitutes Hispanic herbalism. For example, the online class "Traditional Hispanic Herbalism and Magic" covers folklore, wines, teas, vinegars, poultices, and poisons used in the healing process. "Hispanic Materia Medica" includes treatment of specific ailments with native Hispanic Californian and European herbs.

HOLISTIC MEDICINE

Holistic Health is defined by the American Holistic Medical Association as an art and science that treats and prevents disease, while focusing on empowering patients to create a condition of optimal health . . . this state of health is a dynamic balance of the physical, environmental, mental, emotional, social, and spiritual aspects of an individual. As both a healer and health educator, the holistic physician, in partnership with the patient, addresses the causes of disease in addition to treating its symptoms.[1]

Holistic health views environmental, physical, mental, emotional, and spiritual aspects of life as interwoven, so it aims to create balance by attending to all of them. All these aspects must be in sync.

Holistic-online.com
<http://www.holistic-online.com>

Holistic-online.com was created by husband and wife Jacob Mathew, PhD, MBA, and Shila Mathew, MD, a psychiatrist. The Web site features a comprehensive listing of therapies, including humor therapy, color therapy, hydrotherapy, and light therapy. For each therapy, there is a table of conditions or diseases for which the therapy might be used.

HOMEOPATHIC MEDICINE

Homeopathy is the British-based medical practice that treats disease by administering minute doses of natural remedies that would produce the symptoms of the disease in a healthy person, based on the principle "like cures like." The body's own vital force is stimulated to cure itself. Homeopathy is the opposite of allopathic medicine, the most common form of medical practice in the Western world, wherein diseases are treated with

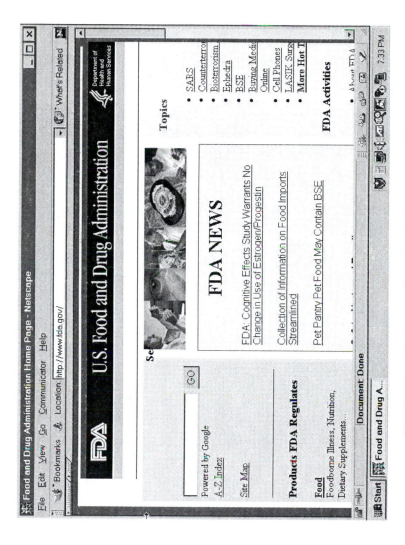

FIGURE 3.7. U.S. Food and Drug Administration Home Page

remedies that produce effects different from those caused by the disease itself.

Homeopathic Educational Services
<http://www.homeopathic.com>

Dana Ullman, who has a master's degree in public health, produces this site. For a fee, the public can obtain a telephone consultation with Ullman. The site provides a very thorough introduction to homeopathy, the FAQ section answers practical questions about the cost of homeopathic care and insurance coverage, and the site sells and publishes books and tapes. See the links under "Specific Ailments and Their Homeopathic Treatment."

Homeopathy Home
<http://www.homeopathyhome.com>

Homeopathy Home includes a directory of homeopathic practitioners, schools, associations, pharmacies, chat rooms, reference materials, Q&A, and services/supplies. There are links to related Web sites. Visitors can purchase books online (in association with Amazon.com).

North American Society of Homeopaths (NASH)
<http://www.homeopathy.org>

NASH's mission is to develop and maintain high standards of homeopathy practice in the United States and Canada. There is a good introduction to homeopathy in the section "How Does Homeopathy Differ from Conventional Medicine?" MDs, DOs, and nutritionists are among its board members. The site includes articles, advice on finding homeopathic practitioners, and lists of schools offering courses in homeopathic medicine.

HUMOR OR CLOWN THERAPY

Association for Applied and Therapeutic Humor (AATH)
<http://www.aath.org>

AATH was founded in 1988. The organization is open to a variety of professions (counselors, doctors, teachers, clergy, social workers, and business executives). This site aims to educate both laymen and health professionals about the value of laughter and humor in health care. Anyone can become a member (for a fee). There are free online articles ("How Can You Laugh at a Time Like This?") and reference lists of published articles for more information.

Carolina Health and Humor Association (HaHa)
<http://www.cahaha.com>

Carolina HaHa is a nonprofit educational service organization founded by Ruth Hamilton, MA Ed. Hamilton is the current executive director. The mission of the organization is to promote a healthy lifestyle through humor and entertainment. Carolina HaHa implemented the Duke University Medical Center's Humor Project. As part of the project, cancer patients use the Laugh Mobile (a mobile display cart designed by Hamilton offering humorous props, books, and tapes). Humor therapy is used to enhance health or provide relief of symptoms of disease. Humor is thought to reduce stress and provide distraction from pain. Click on links to jokes and books for sale. Select "Humor Collection" for information on organizing a humor collection, articles on health and humor, research, health and humor programs, and humor resources.

Gesundheit! Institute (Patch Adams)
<http://patchadams.org>

The mission of the Washington, DC Gesundheit! Institute is "bringing fun, friendship, and the joy of service back into healthcare." Television programs, magazine articles, and a movie have made Dr. Adams well known. The site is geared to health professionals, but anyone can read the online newsletter. Clown therapy and humor are applied to the health care environment.

HUNA

Huna is the Hawaiian word for "secret." The seven Huna principles encompass the power of positive thinking and friendly acceptance of other people and life events. Practitioners try to recognize positive qualities in everyone they meet. Positive energy expended comes back to reward us. Huna practitioners use various relaxation techniques, including positive imaging.

Hawaiian Huna Village
<http://www.huna.org>

This site (see Figure 3.8), sponsored by Aloha International, offers courses and teacher training in the Polynesian spiritual healing techniques known as Huna. Some of the techniques are massage, meditation, dance, chanting, firewalking, and vibrational energy healing. An interesting feature of this site is a link to the **Breast Wishes Institute** (http://www.breastwishes.org), featuring an online support group and other tools to aid women with breast cancer. The focus is on helping patients deal with the rigors of traditional cancer therapy. The site includes recipes, poetry, and meditation. Select "Sharing Hut" to learn about

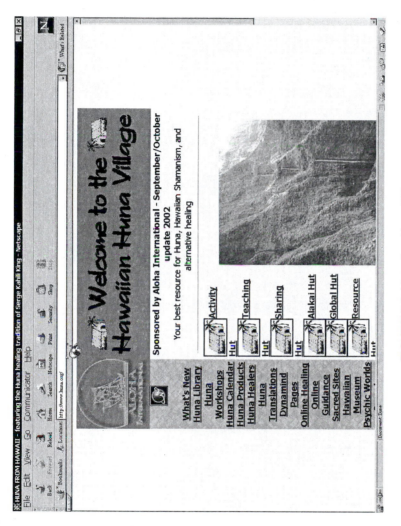

FIGURE 3.8. Hawaiian Huna Village

the weekly online healing circle. Request healing by sending a message to <kaula@aloha.net>. See the Web site for precise instructions. Traditional medical resources (American Cancer Society) and popular books (by Dr. Bernie Siegel, Dr. Susan Love, and Harold Kushner) are also listed. The site lists U.S. and European Huna teachers and therapists.

Huna Kupua
<http://www.hunakupua.com>

Huna Kupua is defined as the "ancient Polynesian system of knowledge and power." In 1979 the passage of the Native American Religious Freedoms Act required Hawaii to abolish all laws banning the practice of Huna. Now it can be freely taught and practiced. This Web site features a very detailed history of Huna.

HYPNOSIS

Hypnosis is the induction of an altered state similar to deep meditation. It is frequently employed to render the patient impervious to pain, as during surgery or dental procedures.

American Society of Clinical Hypnosis (ASCH)
<http://www.asch.net>

ASCH, founded in 1957 by Milton H. Erickson, MD, is the largest organization for health care professionals using clinical hypnosis. This site (see Figure 3.9) provides referrals to hypnosis practitioners. The society's mission is to "encourage and promote excellence in the use of hypnosis by qualified health

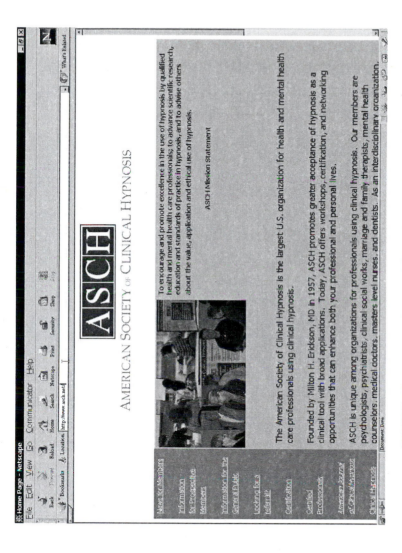

FIGURE 3.9. American Society of Clinical Hypnosis Home Page

and mental health professionals, to advance scientific research, and to advise others about the value, application, and ethical use of hypnosis." There is excellent information on how to select a hypnotherapist. ASCH offers workshops and certification. Select "Information for the General Public" to read a definition of hypnosis and a discussion of the myths about it. The Web site features a list of disorders and symptoms for which hypnosis has applications.

Society for Clinical and Experimental Hypnosis (SCEH)
<http://jceh.wsu.edu/scehframe.htm>

SCEH, founded in 1949, is an international organization of academicians, clinicians, and researchers in fields of medicine, dentistry, nursing, psychology, and social work. SCEH's journal, *International Journal of Clinical and Experimental Hypnosis,* is in many medical school libraries. SCEH emphasizes scientific research and maintains a freely accessible database of thousands of references from journals, books, and scientific meetings. See the section "Hypnosis for the Seriously Curious" which explains the nature of hypnosis, defines the field, tells how to select a hypnotist, and tells what to expect from ethical professional services.

MASSAGE THERAPY

According to the American Massage Therapy Association (AMTA), this is manual soft-tissue manipulation. It includes holding, causing movement, and/or applying pressure to the body. Massage therapy stimulates muscle tissue, creating blood flow through key areas of the body. The increased blood flow is said to help the muscles regenerate.

American Massage Therapy Association
<http://www.amtamassage.org>

This is the official Web site for a national organization representing nearly 50,000 massage therapists in over thirty countries. The organization sets standards, ethics, certification, and school accreditation and offers continuing education courses, lobbies for legislation, and provides public education concerning massage therapy. The site includes links to articles in the professional magazine *Massage Therapy Journal*. This is a good place to locate a certified massage therapist.

NATUROPATHIC THERAPY

Naturopathy aims to restore overall health, rather than suppress a few key symptoms. Practitioners look for the underlying causes of a condition and try to work with the body's natural healing mechanisms. The term "naturopathy" was coined in 1895 by a New Yorker, Dr. John Scheel. Naturopathy includes fasting, acupuncture, massage, herbs, vitamins, and natural food diets.

American Association of Naturopathic Physicians (AANP)
<http://naturopathic.org>

AANP, founded in 1985, is the professional organization of licensed (or eligible for licensing) naturopathic physicians in the United States. This site clearly explains the accreditation process for naturopathic practitioners and aids in the location of local practitioners. The Web site is geared toward naturopathic practitioners, but the FAQs section is excellent for consumers. The association developed standards of practice and was active in promoting the Naturopathic Physicians Licensing Examination (NPLEX).

Association of Natural Medicine Pharmacists (ANMP)
<http://www.anmp.org>

ANMP is a nonprofit professional association of pharmacists and others interested in natural medicines. They offer continuing education courses for members. The Web site's natural medicine question and answer page and herbal quick reference section are useful. Readers can view questions posed by pharmacists and answered by the president of the Association of Natural Medicine Pharmacists. Click on "Monographs" and select "Herbal Quick Reference" for information on kava, ginger, ginseng, and saw palmetto.

Naturopathic Medicine Center
<http://www.healthy.net/clinic/therapy/naturopathic>

The site is produced by HealthWorld Online. The Naturopathic Medicine Center provides very prudent, well-balanced information. See the section "Naturopathic Approach to Specific Health Concerns" (articles written by the American Association of Naturopathic Physicians). Be sure to read "Understanding Natural Medicine." The link "Naturopathic Resource Center" has sections about finding naturopathic practitioners, professional associations, schools, and licensure. The Web site also sells books.

NUTRITION

Nutrition.gov
<http://www.nutrition.gov>

Nutrition.gov (see Figure 3.10) dubs itself "Your guide to nutrition and health information on Federal Government Websites." It is full of useful information with links to many government Web resources. Note the section on dietary supplements, or try searching the keyword "alternative" to retrieve links to diets as alternative treatments for a variety of diseases. There is great material about diabetes and high blood pressure. Nutrition.gov features many bells and whistles on its Web site.

Tufts Nutrition Navigator
<http://navigator.tufts.edu>

Produced by Tufts University Center on Nutrition Communication, this site (see Figure 3.11) features a rating guide to nutrition Web sites. The site describes itself as the "fastest, most reliable way to find sound nutrition information on the Web." Tufts nutritionists evaluate and rate the sites, using criteria developed by the advisory board of Canadian and U.S. nutrition experts. Reviews are arranged by potential users (women, men, seniors, and family). Other categories include general nutrition, weight management, and hot topics.

OSTEOPATHIC MEDICINE

Osteopathy is the medical practice that emphasizes the need to restore the integrity of the body's structure by manipulating its parts. The practice may be supplemented with surgery or administration of drugs.

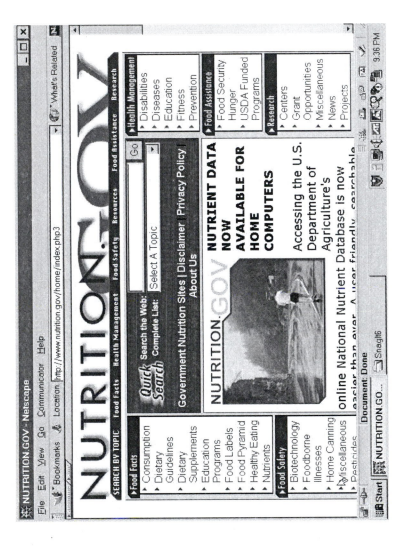

FIGURE 3.10. Nutrition.gov Home Page

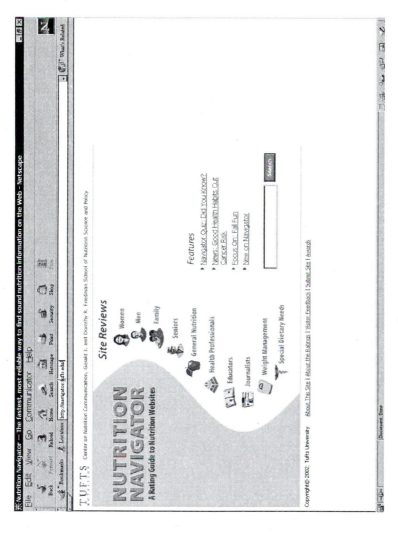

FIGURE 3.11. Tufts Nutrition Navigator Home Page

American Association of Colleges of Osteopathic Medicine (AACOM)
<http://www.aacom.org>

AACOM was founded in 1898. It represents the students, faculty, and administrators of the U.S. colleges of osteopathic medicine. Check out this resource for a good overview of the scope of osteopathic medicine and a history of the field.

The Osteopathic Home Page
<http://www.osteohome.com>

If you have any qualms about consulting an osteopathic physician or you would like to become a DO (Doctor of Osteopathy), this is the site to view (see Figure 3.12). The section "Education" provides details on the training of osteopathic physicians. The site explains that part of the training includes learning when to apply "manual [osteopathic] medicine as a primary treatment" and when to use it as a secondary intervention. Most DOs are on the staff of allopathic as well as osteopathic hospitals. The training of DOs is just as rigorous as that of MDs. The site includes a list of the osteopathic medical schools in the United States. The site explains the nature and history of osteopathy. Why choose an osteopath? How does the body treat itself? Osteopathy views the body as striving toward a healthy balance (homeostasis). The osteopathic practitioner aims to promote this natural healing tendency by a series of body manipulations. A Santa Monica, California, osteopathic physicians group maintains this Web site.

Philadelphia College of Osteopathic Medicine
<http://www.pcom.edu>

In addition to being a good resource to learn about osteopathic medicine, there are some useful CAM links on the library's Web pages: select "Library," then "Internet Guides," and

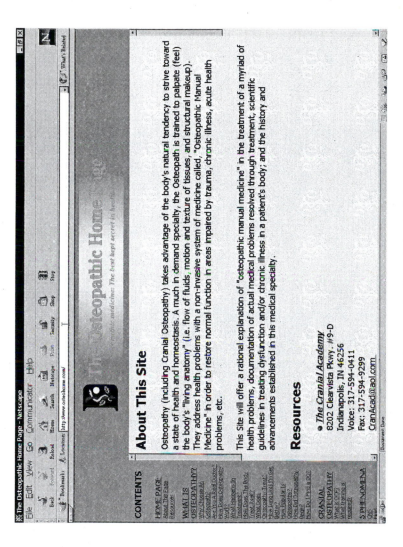

FIGURE 3.12. The Osteopathic Home Page

then "Complementary and Alternative Medicine." The Library's Web pages are packed with many other good medical links. Among the numerous medical school library Web sites, this site stands out for its simplicity.

PET THERAPY

Cats, dogs, and rabbits are frequently scheduled to make calls to patients in hospitals, nursing homes, hospices, and senior centers. Scientific research shows the health benefits of holding, stroking, and walking pets. Organizations certify potential pet therapists by interviewing and testing the animals for gentleness, pleasant personality, obedience, overall health, and appearance. Several organizations certify pet therapists and/or set up pet visitations by their members or outside therapists and their owners.

Delta Society
<http://www.deltasociety.org>

The Delta Society (see Figure 3.13) is one of the best-known organizations of this type. It is an international nonprofit organization espousing the human-animal health connection of "improving human health through service and therapy animals." Read the links under "Health Benefits of Animals." Thanks to a grant from the Geraldine R. Dodge Foundation, the Delta Society is able to include on the site full-text articles and fact sheets documenting the health benefits of animals.

Happy Tails Pet Therapy, Inc.
<http://www.happytailspets.org>

This is an Atlanta-area nonprofit organization. The Web site gives detailed descriptions of the nature of pet-assisted therapy

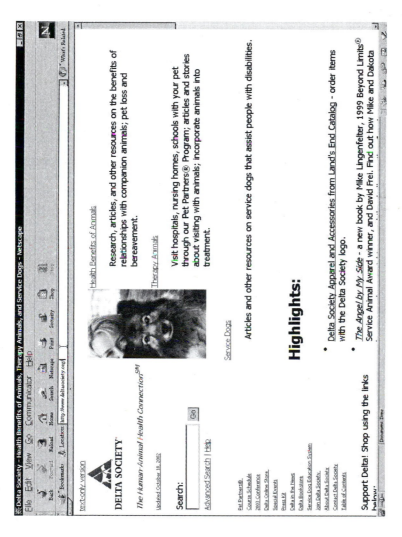

FIGURE 3.13. Delta Society Home Page

93

and explains the different testing requirements for dogs versus cats or other noncanine prospective "therapists." This site is particularly well designed, with plenty of photographs and anecdotes.

Pals for Life
<http://www.palsforlife.org>

Pals for Life is based in suburban Philadelphia. The nonprofit group has been providing pet visitation programs since 1985. The rehabilitation hospital that is part of the health care system where I work schedules regular pet visitation sessions through this organization. Patients gather in a meeting room to pet, brush, and hold a variety of creatures. Afterward, some of the animals visit patients in their rooms. Brushing or petting a dog or cat can help a patient regain range of motion. Depressed, silent patients may open up to a ball of fur, and blood pressure levels may decrease when petting an animal. Click on the links across the top of the home page.

PILATES METHOD

Pilates was developed in Germany in the 1920s by physical therapist Joseph Pilates. The method is an exercise program focused on improving flexibility and strength without producing bulk. Strength training movements are combined with coordinated breathing techniques utilizing special equipment.

The Pilates Studio
<http://www.pilates-studio.com>

The Pilates Studio Web site emphasizes the distinction between a certified Pilates Studio instructor and someone who simply "teaches" Pilates exercises. Pilates includes the use of unique exercise equipment, which can be dangerous if not used correctly. This site helps to locate certified Pilates practitioners and studios. The Web site includes a discussion group.

POLARITY THERAPY

Polarity massage therapy was created in the 1940s by Austrian Dr. Randolph Stone. It is based on the principles of energy and philosophy derived from East Indian Ayurvedic teachings. It is designed to balance the body's electromagnetic energy through touch, stretching exercises, diet, and an emotionally balanced attitude. Its four components are diet, bodywork, movement, and a positive mental attitude.

American Polarity Therapy Association
<http://www.polaritytherapy.org/polarity/>

Polarity therapy was developed by Dr. Randolph Stone, DO, DC, ND, an Austrian immigrant. His first book, *Energy,* was published in 1947. If you are curious about what actually happens during a polarity therapy session, this site gives a detailed description of a typical session. There are many similarities between this technique and Huna, biofeedback, yoga, guided imagery, massage, and osteopathic manipulation. These therapies originated with different cultures, yet they share many core beliefs. Visitors can find a practitioner of polarity therapy at this site.

ROLFING

Rolfing was developed by Dr. Ida Rolf. The formal name is Rolfing Structural Integration. It consists of deep manipulation of the connective tissues ("soft tissues") to relieve misalignment and rigid muscles, joints, and bones. Rolfing is said to improve posture and relieve stress.

Rolf Institute of Structural Integration
<http://www.rolf.org>

The holistic system of soft-tissue manipulation is named for Dr. Ida P. Rolf, a biochemist. She said: "When the body gets working appropriately, the force of gravity can flow through. Then, spontaneously, the body heals itself." The site features a good section on the history of Rolfing. It makes referrals to practitioners in good standing with the institute, which is based in Boulder, Colorado. The institute offers courses leading to certification, as well as continuing education courses.

SHAMANISM

Shamanism is the spiritual and natural healing performed by Native American healers or other members of a tribe or community. Shamans provide healing, advice, and teaching, often by means of altering the state of consciousness of the patient (via meditation, chanting, dancing, smoking, and inhaling or eating psychoactive drugs [certain mushrooms, peyote, herbs, etc.]). Also see the section on Huna in this chapter.

FoxFire Institute of Shamanic Studies
<http://www.foxfireinstitute.com>

FoxFire Institute, based in the United States, Great Britain, and Germany (see Figure 3.14), aims to bridge Western medicine and shamanism, medicine and spirituality. The site contains news, articles, lists of shamanic practitioners, and courses.

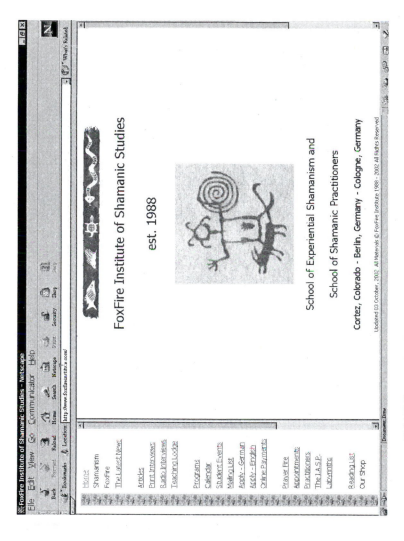

FIGURE 3.14. FoxFire Institute of Shamanic Studies Home Page

There is a weekly "Prayer Fire" service for people in need; e-mail your name, illness or situation, city, state, and country to be included in the prayer circle. The U.S. headquarters is in Cortez, Colorado.

SPIRITUALITY AND PRAYER

Prayer and Spirituality
<http://1stholistic.com/Prayer/hol_prayer_home.htm>

Part of HolisticOnline.com, this site includes the text of popular prayers, arranged by religion. The Web site covers the healing power of prayer, spiritual (including nonreligious) healing, meditation, and yoga. Select links across the top, down the center, and on the left side of the home page.

Spirituality and Health
<http://www.spiritualityhealth.com>

Trinity Church, Wall Street in New York City is the major supporter of this Web site (see Figure 3.15). Spirituality and Health provides explanations of many spiritual beliefs: love, hope, and forgiveness. The site's producers feel there is something "inherently meditative" about using the Internet. They do not think it is strange to have a Web site devoted to spirituality. See the link "Wartime Prayers and Meditations."

VETERINARY CAM

The desire to take medicine is perhaps the greatest feature which distinguishes man from animals.

Sir William Osler (1849-1919)

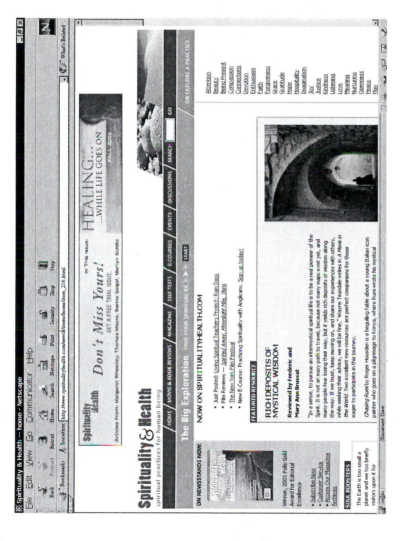

FIGURE 3.15. Spirituality and Health

Academy of Veterinary Homeopathy
<http://www.theavh.org>

The academy is a professional association founded in 1995 by Drs. Pitcairn, Chambreau, and Rygas. Its members include licensed veterinarians and veterinary students who use homeopathy in their practices. The Web site features a referral list of member practitioners who are available for consultations. The academy offers a professional course in veterinary homeopathy. The site includes the "Standards of Practice and Purpose of the Academy."

AltVetMed—Complementary and Alternative Veterinary Medicine
<http://altvetmed.com>

Dr. Jan Agar Bergeron, VMD, established, designed, and maintains the site. Susan Gale Wynn, DVM, is responsible for the content. AltVetMed provides information on CAM in veterinary medicine, including homeopathy, herbs, and nutritional therapy. The site includes a wide variety of links: associations, practitioners, books, supplies, and FAQs. Especially interesting are the links to common problems: "Allergic Skin Disease," "Arthritis," and "Natural Flea Control." Very extensive treatment advice is provided in this section.

Animal Natural Health Center
<http://www.drpitcairn.com>

The center was founded by Richard Pitcairn, DVM, PhD, and emphasizes nutrition, particularly home-prepared and raw foods, sells books and tapes, offers referrals to practitioners, and offers training courses to licensed veterinarians. The text of some of Dr. Pitcairn's lectures is published on the Web site.

Note the alternative advice for cleaning a dog's teeth (select "Health Topics," then "Dentistry Problems for Dogs and Cats").

Holistic Veterinary Medicine: Petsynergy
<http://www.petsynergy.com>

The site covers holistic veterinary care. There are articles, news items, consultations, and bulletin boards (discussion forums). Petsynergy includes directories of acupuncturists and holistic veterinarians.

International Veterinary Acupuncture Society (IVAS)
<http://www.ivas.org>

IVAS's Web site is produced by Dr. Anna Maria Scholey, a Washington State veterinarian. She is certified in veterinary acupuncture and veterinary homeopathy. The site offers referrals to certified veterinary acupuncturists. The society's mission is to be "a worldwide advocate in the promotion of education, responsible research, and the integration of acupuncture into veterinary medicine to create and maintain optimal health in all animals." IVAS is a nonprofit organization that promotes high standards through an accreditation examination and educational programs for veterinarians. The Web site has a message forum and a section on pet astrology. Be sure to read "What Is Veterinary Acupuncture?" for a thorough overview of what it is, how it works, and what conditions are responsive to it.

Tellington Touch (TT)
<http://tteam-ttouch.com>

TT is Linda Tellington-Jones's gentle training/treatment technique for animals, "a training approach for the body, mind, and spirit of animals." TT may be used to assist with recovery from illness or injury. The site includes a worldwide directory of practitioners. Links on the left and right direct visitors to a discussion board, online store, news, TTouch for Dogs and Cats, and TTEAM for Horses. TT is similar to Feldenkrais bodywork. See the section in this chapter on Feldenkrais.

NOTE

1. American Holistic Medical Association. Available at <http://www.holisticmedicine.org>, accessed November 25, 2002.

Chapter 4

CAM for Specific Illnesses
or Symptoms

In addition to the sites listed here, see the Associations/
Organizations section in Chapter 2 for some disease-related
Web sites. **Holistic-Online.com** (http://www.holistic-online.com)
also has a very extensive listing of diseases with suggested
CAM therapies. Included are one or two excellent sites for each
illness. They are a starting point for Internet research.

CANCER

Commonweal
<http://www.commonweal.org>

Commonweal (see Figure 4.1), a small health and environmental research institute located in northern California, aims to
assist patients in making informed decisions about cancer treatment. The information on CAM therapies is thorough and easy
to navigate. Scroll down the home page and click on links of interest. Note the Commonweal Cancer Project and the Commonweal Cancer Help Program. The latter sponsors week-long re-
treats for people with cancer. The Institute for the Study of
Health and Illness is a professional development institute for
physicians.

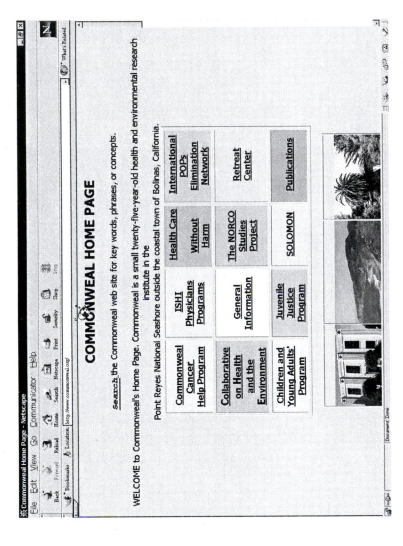

FIGURE 4.1. Commonweal Home Page

OncoLink: Complementary Medicine [for Cancer]
<http://www.oncolink.com/>

OncoLink is very thorough and well documented, and it is updated daily. OncoLink was one of the first high-quality, consumer-oriented medical sites. It has been refined over the years and continues to earn high marks from physicians, nurses, and patients. Select the "Complementary Medicine" section under "Treatment Options." The resource is from the Abramson Cancer Center of the University of Pennsylvania.

CROHN'S DISEASE/COLITIS/ IRRITABLE BOWEL SYNDROME

Crohn's and Colitis Foundation of America (CCFA)
<http://www.ccfa.org>

CCFA's "mission is to cure and prevent Crohn's disease and ulcerative colitis through research, and to improve the quality of life of children and adults affected by these digestive diseases through education and support." Select "Medical Library" and then "Adjunct Therapies." There is a good introduction to the topic of alternative medicine, a discussion of different options, and excellent advice on becoming an educated consumer.

FIBROMYALGIA AND CHRONIC FATIGUE SYNDROME

CFIDS Association of America
<http://www.cfids.org>

CFIDS Association's mission is to conquer the disease. This site (see Figure 4.2) calls the condition chronic fatigue and

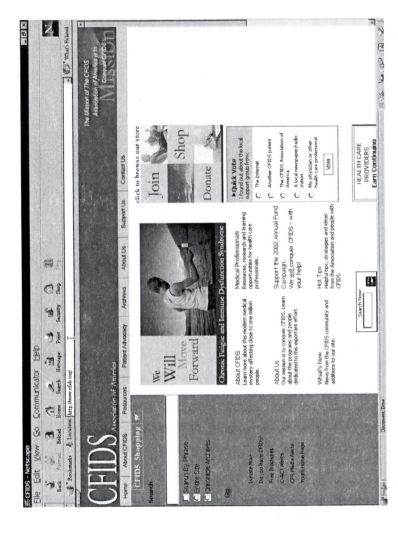

FIGURE 4.2. CFIDS Association of America Home Page. Reprinted by permission of the CFIDS Association of America, Inc.

immune dysfunction syndrome (CFIDS). Select the link "Treatment" and then "Alternative Treatment" for information on the use of therapeutic massage, touch therapy, yoga, and acupuncture in the treatment of this illness. Another section, "Supportive Treatments," lists support groups, disability rights, and advocacy.

Chronic Syndrome Support Association (CSSA)
<http://www.cssa-inc.org>

CSSA, which subscribes to HONcode principles, is a nonprofit organization. It sells a newsletter, books, and tapes, and provides good information about stress and pain management. An interesting and unique feature is a link to **Remedyfind.com** where patients can submit their ratings of various treatments for different conditions. Click on "Multiple Sclerosis" and see patients' opinions of treatments. Other interesting links from the CSSA site cover how to manage housework when experiencing chronic pain, discussion groups, Gulf War syndrome, fibromyalgia, multiple chemical sensitivities syndrome, and other chronic immunological and neurological disorders.

ImmuneSupport.com
<http://www.immunesupport.com>

This is a commercial Web site, but it contains many links to resources about chronic, debilitating conditions such as fibromyalgia and chronic fatigue syndrome. The site also has links to message boards and support groups.

HEPATITIS C

Hepatitis C: Treatment Alternatives
<http://nccam.nih.gov/health/hepatitisc>

This is a page on the Web site of the National Center for Complementary and Alternative Medicine. The center states that alternative medicine cannot cure hepatitis C, but alternative treatments may help patients cope with side effects of the disease and its medical treatment. The site has a rating scale (0 through 3) for treatments based on the amount of rigorous scientific research that exists for a particular therapy. A rating of 0 means no research exists because no scientific studies have been done. A rating of 3 means extensive research exists, based on clinical trials with human patients, and the results have been published in reputable medical journals. Milk thistle and licorice root are two of the plants discussed at length.

MENOPAUSE

Menopause Online
<http://www.menopause-online.com/treatments.htm>

"Devoted to providing women with up-to-date information," this site is sponsored by ThirdAge, Inc. and consists of a Web site, membership, and an affinity group for baby boomers (those born between 1946 and 1964). Menopause Online clearly discusses and distinguishes between traditional and alternative treatments for unpleasant symptoms that often accompany this transition. The site also features a bulletin board for online discussions and subscribes to the HONcode principles of the Health on the Net Foundation. Menopause Online compares favorably with the Web site of the North American Menopause Society, but the latter site is geared more to physicians.

North American Menopause Society (NAMS)
<http://www.menopause.org>

NAMS is a scientific nonprofit organization "promoting women's health during midlife and beyond through an understanding of menopause." NAMS's Web site has sections for health professionals (members and nonmembers) and consumers. It follows the HONcode principles and is very up to date. Note the section "Alternatives to Hormones." Click on the segment for consumers and browse the links. There is a menopause discussion list and directories of NAMS member clinicians (physicians and nurses) in the United States and Canada.

MULTIPLE SCLEROSIS (MS)

National Multiple Sclerosis Society
<http://www.nationalmssociety.org>

The National Multiple Sclerosis Society is an organization with local chapters providing advocacy, support, education, and promotion of research. This is a fine example of a well-balanced, up-to-date medical Web site that provides thoughtful, well-documented material on complementary therapies along with traditional treatments. Select "Treatments" then "Therapies—Alternative." Be sure to read the sections "Clear Thinking About Alternative Therapies," "Understanding Your Options," and "Please Be Careful." A patient wrote the last section; she discusses the feelings of desperation and vulnerability that confront people with serious chronic illnesses. For in-depth information on CAM, there is a link to **MS-CAM** (http://www.

ms-cam.org), produced by the Rocky Mountain MS Center in Colorado. See the section for newly diagnosed MS patients.

PARKINSON'S DISEASE

Complementary Therapies and Parkinson's Disease
<http://www.parkinson.org/therapies.htm>

This is a section on the National Parkinson Foundation (NPF) Web site. NPF's mission is to find a cure for Parkinson's disease and related neurodegenerative diseases through research. NPF also aims to educate physicians, the public, and patients and their caregivers and to improve the quality of life of patients and their caregivers. The Web site is very thorough and well balanced. See the section written by two physicians on staff at two National Parkinson Foundation Centers of Excellence. They explain ways that CAM therapies such as massage, yoga, herbal medicine, acupuncture, and coenzyme Q10 can complement standard drug therapy of this disease.

Emory University Center for Research on Complementary and Alternative Medicine in Neurodegenerative Diseases
<http://www.emory.edu/WHSC/MED/NEUROLOGY/CAM/index.html>

The center conducts systematic research on CAM for patients with Parkinson's disease, Alzheimer's disease, multiple sclerosis, stroke, and Huntington's disease. It is one of the dozen CAM centers funded by NCCAM. There is a listing of opportunities for patients to participate in research studies and a segment on the center's current research projects. One project is "Chinese exercise modalities in Parkinson's disease." The site provides links to several general CAM Web sites. There is also a section on neurodegenerative disease Web resources.

SICKLE-CELL DISEASE

Sickle Cell Disease Association of America (SCDAA)
<http://www.sicklecelldisease.org>

SCDAA was founded over thirty years ago. Over the years they have produced workshops, issued educational materials, and offered counseling programs and screening services. They underwrite grants supporting research at Comprehensive Sickle Cell Centers. The site includes chat room forums: family support, Q&A, and peer support. There is no segment specific to CAM at the Web site, but visitors can pose questions related to sickle-cell disease and CAM on the discussion forum.

Chapter 5

Parting Advice:
Ready, Set, "Google"

You've read the book, explored some Web sites, and lurked in some chat rooms or newsgroups. Now what? Here are some suggestions:

1. Set up a personal filing system on your home computer. Depending upon the Internet service provider, the files may be called "bookmarks" or "favorites," or marked with hearts in a virtual file cabinet. Basically, you will select Web sites you want to visit regularly and set them aside in folders. You can set up broad categories to group related sites together in one folder. For example, if you have a spouse and children, you might want to create folders for each of them. In "Ben's folder" you could put your favorite Web sites for CAM treatment of arthritis and headaches. In "Grandma's folder," place the Web sites for CAM and menopause and CAM and colitis. In "Mom's folder," keep the Web addresses for sites useful for CAM and women's health issues. In "Suzy's folder," bookmark sites on CAM and attention deficit disorder/hyperactivity. You can create folders for the Internet addresses of newsgroups and bulletin boards, for favorite search engines, and for favorite general gateway CAM resources at university library Web sites.
2. Experiment with the search engines. See what sites you find that are relevant to your specific interests.

3. Create a personalized subset of the resources described in this book. Choose one or two sites from each chapter. Use these frequently. Become an expert in finding information on these sites.
4. Above all, relax and enjoy the anonymity and variety of the Internet.
5. Do not forget to discuss your search results with your doctor or nurse *before* you try out any therapies.

Glossary

acupuncture: The traditional Chinese practice of puncturing the skin in precise locations with fine needles in order to cure diseases or to relieve pain. It was developed more than 3,000 years ago and is based on Taoist philosophy. It aims to balance the energy meridians to allow the body to heal itself.

Alexander technique: AT was developed in the 1890s by F. Alexander, an Australian actor. Practitioners use gentle touch and observation to change the body's patterns of movement. A goal is reeducating the patient to change poor habits of coordination. Practitioners of the technique believe habits of excessive tension and inefficient coordination affect how one feels and thinks. The technique focuses on correct posture and the correct way to lift objects.

allopathic medicine: A method of treating diseases with remedies that produce effects different from those caused by the disease itself. This is the most common form of medical practice in the Western world.

aromatherapy: The topical or inhaled application of botanical oils (essential oils) extracted from barks, flowers, grasses, and herbs. Examples are lemon oil, sage, eucalyptus oil, and sandalwood. Aromatherapy is an ancient healing art that dates back to 4500 B.C.

Ayurvedic medicine/Ayurveda: The traditional Indian, nature-based health care aimed at achieving a state of balance between body and mind. Ayurveda offers multiple strategies for harmonizing mind, body, and spirit through herbs, diet, meditation, massage, aromatherapy, and self-healing regimens.

chiropractic care: This employs manipulation and adjustment of body structures (particularly the spine) to cure diseases through the restoration of normal nerve function. Chiropractic is commonly used to treat backache, chronic pain, and poor posture.

complementary and alternative medicine (CAM): Treatments and health care practices not taught widely in medical schools, not generally used in hospitals, and not generally reimbursed by medical insurance companies.

Feldenkrais work: Feldenkrais includes the principles developed by Moshe Feldenkrais and is based on physics and biomechanics. It employs gentle movement to gradually increase range of motion, flexibility, balance, and coordination. Feldenkrais attempts to reprogram the nervous system by means of movement supplemented by physical pressure and manipulation.

guided imagery (GI): The process of imaging through any of the senses (taste, touch, smell, hearing, and sight). Examples are biofeedback, hypnosis, desensitization, relaxation techniques, and transcendental meditation). GI often involves listening to music or a person's voice in a relaxed setting, so imagery and deep feelings can surface from one's inner self.

herbalism: The practice of applying or administering specific herbs to treat medical problems.

holistic health: This is defined by the American Holistic Medical Association as "an art and science that treats and prevents disease, while focusing on empowering patients to create a condition of optimal health. . . . [T]his state of health is a dynamic balance of the physical, environmental, mental, emotional, social, and spiritual aspects of an individual. As both a healer and health educator, the holistic physician, in partnership with the patient, addresses the causes of disease in addition to treating its symptoms" (available at <http://www.holistic medicine.org>, accessed November 25, 2002). Holistic health views environmental, physical, mental, emotional and spiritual aspects of life as interwoven, so it aims to create balance by attending to all. All these aspects must be in sync.

holistic medicine: A general term for various forms of complementary and alternative medicine.

homeopathy: Homeopathy is the British-based medical practice that treats disease by administering minute doses of natural remedies that would produce the symptoms of the disease in a healthy person. "Like cures like." The body's own vital force is stimulated to cure itself.

Huna: Polynesian shamanism. *See also* SHAMANISM.

hypnosis: Hypnosis is the induction of an altered state similar to deep meditation. It is frequently employed to render the patient impervious to pain, as during surgery or dental procedures.

integrative medicine: "[B]rings together conventional medical care with promising alternative approaches to healing . . . to offer a coordinated, expanded approach to healthcare." It uses whatever methods are most effective, without favoring one system over another (traditional or alternative). Integrative medicine does not put down traditional (Western) medicine (Thomas Jefferson University Hospital—Center for Integrative Medicine, available at <http://Jeffersonhospital.org>, accessed January 2003).

massage therapy: According to the American Massage Therapy Association, this is manual soft-tissue manipulation. It includes holding, causing movement, and/or applying pressure to the body.

Native American traditional healing: Local herbal remedies, shamans, sweat lodges, and healing ceremonies.

naturopathic medicine/naturopathy: Aims to restore overall health, rather than suppress a few key symptoms. Practitioners look for the underlying causes of a condition and try to work with the body's natural healing mechanisms. The term *naturopathy* was first coined in 1895 by a New Yorker, Dr. John Scheel. Naturopathy includes fasting, acupuncture, massage, herbs, vitamins, and natural food diets.

osteopathic medicine/osteopathy: The medical practice that emphasizes the need to restore the integrity of the body's structure by manipulating its parts. The practice may be supplemented with surgery or administration of drugs.

Pilates method: Pilates was developed in Germany in the 1920s by physical therapist Joseph Pilates. The method is an exercise program focused on improving flexibility and strength without producing bulk. Strength-training movements are combined with coordinated breathing techniques, utilizing special equipment.

polarity massage therapy: Polarity massage therapy was created in the 1900s by Austrian Dr. Randolph Stone. It is based on the principles of energy and philosophy derived from East Indian Ayurvedic teachings. It is designed to balance the body's electromagnetic energy through touch, stretching exercises, diet, and an emotionally balanced attitude. Its four components include diet, body work, movement, and a positive mental attitude.

reflexology: The ancient Chinese technique employing pressure point massage (usually of the feet) to restore flow of energy throughout the body.

Rolfing: Rolfing was developed by Dr. Ida Rolf. The formal name is Rolfing Structural Integration. It consists of deep manipulation of the connective tissues ("soft tissues") in order to relieve misalignment and rigid muscles, joints, and bones. Rolfing is said to improve posture and relieve stress.

shamanism: The spiritual and natural healing performed by Native American medicine men or other members of a tribe or community. Shamans provide healing, advice, and teaching, often by means of altering the state of consciousness of the patient (via meditation, chanting, dancing, smoking, inhaling, or eating psychoactive plants [certain mushrooms, peyote, herbs, etc.]). *See also* HUNA.

sweat lodge: The ancient Native American body purification ceremony involving use of intense heat, similar to that of a sauna, to provoke insights and visions.

tai chi: The Chinese Taoist martial arts form of meditation in movement, combining mental concentration, coordinated breathing, and a sense of slow, graceful body movements. It is a form of mobile meditation used for relaxation, balance, self-defense, and reenergizing.

Tellington Touch or Ttouch (TT): Ttouch is Linda Tellington-Jones's training and treatment system for animals. The method is based on Feldenkrais work, the application of circular movements of the hands and fingers over the entire body. It is said to activate cellular function.

visualization: Similar to light hypnosis, visualization creates a soothing environment for relaxation and aids one to overcome phobias and other problems.

yoga: Yoga is the ancient Hindu system of stretching and toning the body through movements and postures. It improves flexibility, muscle tone, and mobility.

Index

Page numbers followed by the letter "f" indicate figures.

SPECIAL 25%-OFF DISCOUNT!

Order a copy of this book with this form or online at:

http://www.haworthpress.com/store/product.asp?sku=4986

THE GUIDE TO COMPLEMENTARY AND ALTERNATIVE MEDICINE ON THE INTERNET

_____in hardbound at $22.46 (regularly $29.95) (ISBN: 0-7890-1570-6)

_____in softbound at $11.21 (regularly $14.95) (ISBN: 0-7890-1571-4)

Or order online and use special offer code HEC25 in the shopping cart.

COST OF BOOKS_____

OUTSIDE US/CANADA/
MEXICO: ADD 20%_____

POSTAGE & HANDLING_____
*(US: $5.00 for first book & $2.00
for each additional book)*
Outside US: $6.00 for first book)
& $2.00 for each additional book)

SUBTOTAL_____

IN CANADA: ADD 7% GST_____

STATE TAX_____
*(NY, OH MN, CA, IN, & SD residents,
add appropriate local sales tax)*

FINAL TOTAL_____
*(If paying in Canadian funds,
convert using the current
exchange rate, UNESCO
coupons welcome)*

Prices in US dollars and subject to change without notice.

☐ **BILL ME LATER:** ($5 service charge will be added)
(Bill-me option is good on US/Canada/Mexico orders only;
not good to jobbers, wholesalers, or subscription agencies.)

☐ Check here if billing address is different from
shipping address and attach purchase order and
billing address information.

Signature_____

☐ **PAYMENT ENCLOSED: $**_____

☐ **PLEASE CHARGE TO MY CREDIT CARD.**

☐ Visa ☐ MasterCard ☐ AmEx ☐ Discover
☐ Diner's Club ☐ Eurocard ☐ JCB

Account #_____

Exp. Date_____

Signature_____

NAME_____

INSTITUTION_____

ADDRESS_____

CITY_____

STATE/ZIP_____

COUNTRY_____ COUNTY (NY residents only)_____

TEL_____ FAX_____

E-MAIL_____

May we use your e-mail address for confirmations and other types of information? ☐ Yes ☐ No
We appreciate receiving your e-mail address and fax number. Haworth would like to e-mail or fax special
discount offers to you, as a preferred customer. **We will never share, rent, or exchange your e-mail address
or fax number.** We regard such actions as an invasion of your privacy.

Order From Your Local Bookstore or Directly From

The Haworth Press, Inc.

10 Alice Street, Binghamton, New York 13904-1580 • USA

TELEPHONE: 1-800-HAWORTH (1-800-429-6784) / Outside US/Canada: (607) 722-5857

FAX: 1-800-895-0582 / Outside US/Canada: (607) 771-0012

E-mailto: orders@haworthpress.com

PLEASE PHOTOCOPY THIS FORM FOR YOUR PERSONAL USE.

http://www.HaworthPress.com

BOF03